W9-DCE-612

Security

Keeping the Health Care Environment Safe

Russell L. Colling, MS, CHPA, CPP

Joint Commission Mission   The mission of the Joint Commission on Accreditation of Healthcare Organizations is to improve the quality of care provided to the public through the provision of health care accreditation and related services that support performance improvement.

Joint Commission educational programs and publications support, but are separate from, the accreditation activities of the Joint Commission. Attendees at Joint Commission educational programs and purchasers of Joint Commission publications receive no special consideration or treatment in, or confidential information about, the accreditation process.

© 1996 by the Joint Commission on Accreditation of Healthcare Organizations
One Renaissance Boulevard Oakbrook Terrace, IL 60181

All rights reserved. No part of this book may be reproduced in any form or by any means without written permission from the publisher.

Printed in the U.S.A.   5   4   3   2   1

Requests for permission to reprint or make copies of any part of this work should be mailed to:
Permissions Editor
Department of Publications
Joint Commission on Accreditation of Healthcare Organizations
One Renaissance Boulevard
Oakbrook Terrace, IL 60181

http://www.jcaho.org

ISBN: 0–86688–469–6

Library of Congress Catalog Card Number: 96–077406

HELP US MEET YOUR NEEDS.

We'd like your opinion of Security: *Keeping the Health Care Environment Safe.* Your input will help us improve the quality of this and other publications. Please—take just a moment to complete and return this card.

If you'd like more information about Joint Commission publications, please call Customer Service at 630-792-5800.

What did you find most/least useful about this book?

Most useful:

_____

_____

Least useful:

_____

_____

What improvements would you suggest for this book?

_____

_____

_____

What other topics/types of publications would you like to see produced to meet your Environment of Care needs?

_____

_____

Additional comments:

_____

_____

Your title: _____

Type and size of organization:_____

Name/Address (optional):

_____

_____

Thank you!

BUSINESS REPLY MAIL

FIRST CLASS MAIL   PERMIT NO 632   VILLA PARK IL

POSTAGE WILL BE PAID BY ADDRESSEE

JOINT COMMISSION ON ACCREDITATION
OF HEALTHCARE ORGANIZATIONS
ONE RENAISSANCE BOULEVARD
OAKBROOK TERRACE IL   60181-9887
ATTN KRISTINE TOMASIK

NO POSTAGE
NECESSARY IF
MAILED IN THE
UNITED STATES

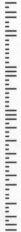

*"A management plan
addresses security."*

*—The Comprehensive Accreditation Manual
for Hospitals,*

*The Joint Commission
on Accreditation of Healthcare Organizations*

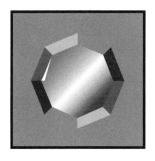

Security: Keeping the Health Care Environment Safe

by Russell L. Colling, MS, CHPA, CPP

About the Author: **Russell L. Colling, MS, CHPA, CPP,** is a recognized lecturer, seminar presenter, and consultant in the field of health care security. The founder of the International Association for Healthcare Security and Safety (IAHSS), Mr Colling has more than 25 years experience in the health care security field. He is currently Executive Vice President-Security for Hospital Shared Services of Colorado, in Denver.

We also wish to thank the following people for their help in making this book possible:

Writer: **Lauren Phillips** has written numerous articles, books, and newsletters for a variety of health care and other clients.

Reviewers:

Errol Biggs, PhD, is Director, the Center for Health Administration, the University of Colorado at Denver.

Bonnie Michelman, CPP, CHPA, is Director of Police and Security at Massachusetts General Hospital, Boston, and President, International Association for Healthcare Security and Safety.

Thomas A. Scaletta, MD, FACEP, is Associate Director, Department of Emergency Medicine, Cook County Hospital, Chicago; Associate Professor of Emergency Medicine, Rush Medical College, Chicago; and Midwest Regional Coordinator, Physicians for a Violence-Free Society.

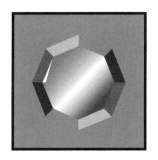

Contents

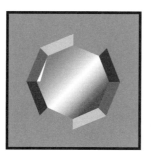

A Foreword from the Occupational Safety and Health Administration (OSHA)

According to the Bureau of Labor Statistics, almost two thirds of nonfatal assaults are occurring in service industries such as nursing homes, hospitals, and establishments providing residential care and other social services. These assaults are primarily by patients on nursing staff in health care institutions. The mission of the Occupational Safety and Health Administration (OSHA) is to protect the safety and health of American workers. Accordingly, OSHA released a set of voluntary guidelines on March 14, 1996, to prevent workplace violence for health care and social service workers.

The guidelines cover a broad spectrum of workers in psychiatric facilities, hospital emergency departments, community mental health clinics, drug treatment clinics, pharmacies, community care facilities, and long-term care facilities. Nearly 8 million workers are covered by the new guidelines, including physicians, registered nurses, pharmacists, nurse practitioners, physician assistants, nurses' aides, therapists, technicians, public health nurses, home health workers, social/welfare workers, and emergency medical care personnel.

Hundreds of lawsuits are filed each year against health care institutions for failure to provide proper security protection. There are many known risk factors in today's health care facilities that are described in OSHA's guidelines, as well as in this book. While health care facilities can't predict or avoid all incidents, a sound protection program can lessen the impact and reduce the odds.

OSHA's guidelines contain four main components that are recommended for an effective safety and health program: (1) management commitment and employee involvement, (2) worksite analysis, (3) hazard prevention and control, and (4) safety and health training.

Management commitment and employee involvement are needed in the establishment and implementation of a performance measurement system in which various safeguards are applied to each security risk and a specified outcome for each safeguard assigned. The health care organization should establish what is, and is not, acceptable, i.e., an acceptable threshold or risk tolerance level. There should be a quantitative analysis of risk levels and risk probability reduced to a practical and realistic level. Commitment to the overall mission of the organization, including good security, is required of all personnel, whether management, caregiver, or security.

The formal risk assessment (also referred to as a needs identification or security survey), serves as the worksite analysis. The objective of the risk assessment is to thoroughly examine every function and physical space in the organization in order to identify and quantify the security risk exposure, particularly in security-sensitive areas. The assessment involves a review of data and reports, a review of staff input, and a hands-on inspection. Standards should spell out specific requirements for safeguarding areas designated as security sensitive, such as: ED/ICU's, maternity and infant care, pharmacy, parking, and facility-specific security areas, such as medical records, cashiers, medical research, and mental health care.

For hazard prevention and control, all types of physical security should be addressed and analyzed, i.e., metal detectors, locks, lighting (ANSI standards), fencing and other barriers, signage, glazing, security officers, integrated systems approach (closed-circuit television, electronic digital key pad or card readers, video recorders, alarm systems), and security through environmental design (Crime Prevention Through Environmental Design–CPTED). It is emphasized, as in the OSHA guidelines, that the need to implement security measures will vary with each establishment according to the risk factors identified. The security management plan for a specific establishment will also change based upon the ongoing risk assessment process. Administrative and work practice controls are also helpful; examples are flagging records of violent patients and interventions as a response to crisis (verbal, social, pharmacologic, and physical).

Finally, training is required in basic security practices, particularly in security sensitive areas. Training in the use of policies and procedures is advocated with the roles and expectations of participants carefully defined and communicated. Employees should receive training when first hired and as an ongoing management process. Types of training are: basic pre-assignment training, pre-post assignment training, periodic in-service training, skills training, and staff development.

Maintenance of records and reports is also important. Incident reports are crucial to performing a security risk assessment and for ongoing modifications and changes to the security management plan. The similarities to OSHA's guidelines are many, and this book serves a valuable purpose as a supplemental tool to these guidelines for health care establishments that seek to provide a safe and secure environment for employees and patients.

—**Joseph A. Dear**
   Assistant Secretary, OSHA
—**Patricia Biles**
   Workplace Violence Program Coordinator, OSHA

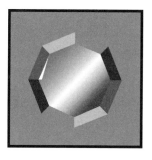

Introduction

"71-year-old surgery patient opens fire in Arizona hospital."

"Infant kidnapped from California hospital nursery."

"IV tubes slashed in Florida ICU."

These alarming headlines offer just a glimpse of the serious security situation facing every health care facility in the United States today. No facility can be made totally safe. But all can be made reasonably secure through a managed system of safeguards designed to protect property and achieve relative safety for everyone within the immediate environment.

This handbook offers a comprehensive, down-to-earth approach to designing and operating such a system in any health care facility, regardless of location, size, or type—inner city research institute, rural community hospital, or suburban medical center. In addition to serving as a quick reference guide to the basic functions and principles of health care security, it provides a solid foundation of information on which to build security plans and programs that meet all current legal and regulatory standards of practice.

The incidence of workplace violence in the health care setting continues to grow in tandem with the incidence of violence in the American workplace in general. A recent study by the Northwestern National Life Insurance Company revealed that 25% of full-time U.S. workers were harassed, threatened, or attacked while on the job within the previous 12 months; among those who dealt directly with the public, that figure was 50%. Annually, this translates to more than two million physical attacks on workers.[1] Among nurses, 76% say they have been assaulted at least once in their career.[2] Clearly, violence in the workplace is responsible for a great deal of human suffering. It also has a tremendous impact on the cost of delivering health care, not just through lost productivity and medical treatment of the injured, but through property losses and litigation as well.

Acts of dishonesty—theft, pilferage, kickbacks, sabotage, damage planned coolly or carried out in the heat of rage, and outright waste—are perpetrated by staff, patients, and visitors to health care facilities. But the employee inflicts the greatest property loss in any organization. Health care workers, in particular, are exposed to a wealth of supplies and equipment that are both useful in the home and readily salable on the open market. Moving even bulky items is made easier given the relative freedom to come and go at all hours most such workers have.

As for lawsuits, hundreds are filed every year against health care organizations for failing to provide proper security protection. Most such cases of "premises liability litigation" involve allegations that the organization either did not act or acted negligently in performing its duty to protect. To the enormous cost of defending such suits, including settlements or court awards, must be added the less tangible but no less real harm caused the organization by adverse publicity and its effects on staff.

Caregivers who fear their patients and their patients' visitors can hardly perform at their peak. And this fear goes far beyond the time of actual treatment, as revealed in reports of stalking and harassment of health care employees outside the work environment. There are countless reports of serious injury, even murder, to health care workers, by former patients or family members who have harbored resentment for years after what they perceived to be a bad health care experience.

Although all persons on the property of the organization, including visitors, are exposed to security risks, none are more vulnerable than the patients. Their age, medical condition and/or treatment may render them unable to fully comprehend their surroundings or to contribute to their own safety.

This exposure, this vulnerability, is a constant in today's health care facility, regardless of how sheltered it may appear to be by virtue of its geographic location, demographics, or history. For this reason, it is essential that hospitals take a proactive stance toward security. In too many places, only after a violent incident are steps taken to prevent a recurrence.

Good business sense dictates that, instead of waiting for a crisis to arise, every organization that has not already done so should act now to erect a strong security barrier between itself and those who would do it harm.

The first step is a formal risk assessment, described in detail in Chapter 2. Sometimes called a needs identification or security survey, this is the start of a management program cycle called for by Joint Commission Environment of Care standards. The cycle includes plan design, implementation, measurement and assessment, and improvement; the ongoing process is identical to that used for many other business activities within the health care organization.

The design step is one of applying security safeguards to properly manage the risks identified in the assessment. The major task in the implementation phase is training and educating staff members, including the user and/or the provider of each safeguard, along with ordering and installing equipment.

Measurement and assessment begin immediately upon implementation, with fine-tuning procedures and equipment, making minor modifications in design or training, and using measurement instruments, including incident reports, to evaluate the safeguards' effectiveness. These processes are examined in Part II.

The security management plan is dynamic, not static. Minor shifts will occur as the organizational structure and physical environment change; major changes will take place as dictated by shortfalls in intended outcomes. In some cases, the needs or risks themselves may change, at which point the design phase is revisited and the entire cycle begun again.

Organizations that have such a security program in place should take this opportunity to review and rethink each plan component to ensure that they are capable of meeting every conceivable challenge—not just those likely to occur or those that have occurred before. Special attention should be paid to those areas of the organization designated "security sensitive," the subject of Part III.

Readers may want to think of the principles and practices described in this book, grounded in more than three decades of real-world experience, as a special kind of safety net: flexible enough to accommodate every kind of health care organization but sturdy enough to protect those inside who need care—and those who do the caring.

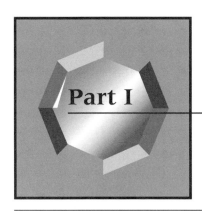

Part I

Security and the Health Care Environment

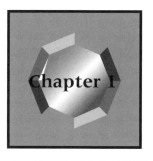

Chapter 1

The Health Care Organization as a Unique Security Challenge

In the not-too-distant past, hospitals, like churches, were thought to be something of a safe haven, relatively free from common crime. Today the medical care facility is fair game for all the ills of society, from murder and arson to the sometimes petty disruptions of disgruntled visitors, patients, and staff. Maintaining a reasonably safe and secure environment in today's world requires a serious commitment by the health care organization.

■ *What Security Is, and Is Not*

This book defines security as the establishment of a system of safeguards designed to protect physical property and to achieve relative safety for all people within the organization and its environment.*

One of the most troubling misconceptions about security is that it is synonymous with law enforcement. Although their goals and objectives overlap, their activities and functions are, for the most part, vastly different. Security is, first and foremost, a

---

*As used here, the term safety is more inclusive than security. An accidental needle stick or a fall on a wet floor is a safety problem and not a security risk. So while the director of security would most likely sit on the hospital's environment of care of (as it used to be known) safety committee, security would only be one item on the committee's agenda.

proactive force, geared toward prevention of wrongdoing. Law enforcement, on the other hand, is a reactive force, geared toward apprehension of the wrongdoer. (See Figure 1.1.) The distinction can be troubling for police officers turned security guards, which is why many experienced hospital security chiefs steer clear of what might seem to be an obvious source of personnel.

In addition to being protective, health care security also may be seen as service-oriented, contributing to and supporting the organization's overall mission. In fact, the scope, direction, and activities of the security program should directly reflect the organization's stated aims. For example, if a hospital is committed to fostering the research activities of an affiliated medical school, then its security program may encompass the protection of the researchers and their work—including, in many cases, research involving animals (which may arouse a different kind of protective instinct among some violence-prone activists).

SECURITY VS LAW ENFORCEMENT:
General Characteristics

Security	Law Enforcement
Proactive	Reactive
Prevention	Apprehension
General Services	Prosecution
Defined by Organization	Defined by Statute
Protect an Organization	Protect a Society
Private Funding	Tax Supported

Figure 1.1. *Law enforcement and security are not synonymous, but complementary, forces.*

Security must permeate the entire organization. It must be—
and must be perceived as—an integral part of its everyday life. In
this respect, security is not isolated: In addition to their primary
responsibilities, hospital staff at all levels must accept the need to
practice good security at all times.

Everything said up to this point could also be said of a security program at a manufacturing plant, sporting event, airport,
bank, or used car lot. But while security principles and systems
everywhere are, to a certain extent, alike, it is their application in
a specific setting that determines a successful program. Security
in a health care organization is unique because the health care
organization itself is unique. (See Figure 1.2.)

■ Unique Security Considerations

A modern medical center is essentially an open campus. It runs
24 hours a day, typically offering walk-in emergency services the
entire time, with only limited restrictions on public access.

**UNIQUE ENVIRONMENTAL FACTORS AFFECTING HOSPITAL
SECURITY**

High stress levels/emotionally charged atmosphere

In operation 24 hours a day

Open environment

Continuous shift changes

Large numbers of technical staff

Large numbers of female staff

Figure 1.2. *A hospital is a place where very private business is conducted
in a very public manner—an often volatile mix.*

Although there has been some movement recently toward a return to visitor pass systems, marketing efforts over the last two decades have been directed toward creating a user-friendly atmosphere to counter the loss of inpatient census.

The medical center operates at a high participant stress level: The patients are obviously stressed, the caregivers at times only slightly less so. Interestingly, the stress of the visitors, which might at first be considered secondary, is a factor of great importance in securing the environment.

Persons who are not patients or staff members fall into one of two categories—legitimate or illegitimate visitors, each of which presents its own problems. Legitimate visitors may erupt out of frustration and anxiety, usually connected with a patient whose treatment they perceive to be inadequate or inappropriate. Disrespect for rules, regulations, other patients, and staff activities can exacerbate such acting out, a situation that arises most often when large numbers of people visit a single patient—for example, a group of gang members visiting a fellow member.

The illegitimate visitor—imposter, sneak thief, assaulter, defacer of property, stalker, hostage taker, kidnapper, arsonist—will blend in with the legitimate visitors to an often remarkable degree. Given the potential for such persons to wreak havoc, we can consider ourselves lucky that the opportunity and intent to commit such criminal acts only rarely coincide in our hospital corridors.

The increasing popularity of 12-hour shifts means that technical staff are coming and going at all hours of the night. And many of these people, not just physicians, are often preoccupied with life-and-death situations, making them less alert and less likely to follow good security practices. It has long been recognized that staff are vulnerable to assaults in parking lots, particularly during off-hours, but more so when persons are reporting for work (which they tend to do singly rather than in groups) and leaving late. Although a security escort service is provided by most organizations, the employee finishing work is often in a hurry and resists waiting to be escorted. An escort service for arriving employees is virtually impossible to provide.

Actually, it is the visitor, less likely overall to be the victim of crime than either staff member or patient, who is most likely to run into trouble on the grounds outside the facility. Statistics reveal that more staff members are assaulted or killed in their work areas than outside, most often by disgruntled patients, unhappy coworkers, or domestic partners. Staff working alone in remote areas are at special risk.

The organization itself is exposed to a multitude of risks, the most common of which is the theft or destruction of property. Loss, improper use, disclosure, and manipulation of information is also a real threat to proper functioning. A northern Florida hospital recently was the victim of a prank by a teenage daughter of a staff member. While visiting her mother, who was on duty, the teenager accessed a computer file listing persons who had been treated over the weekend in the emergency department. She called seven of these patients, telling them they were infected with HIV; one call was to the mother of a teenager, who was told her daughter was not only HIV positive but pregnant as well.

Of course, the degree of risk varies from facility to facility. Although all hospital cashier functions, for example, are subject to the risk of armed robbery, the inner-city facility that handles large amounts of cash and is open for business 16 hours a day faces a high degree of risk compared to a small, rural facility that handles little cash and has restricted hours. On the other hand, a rural facility may face a greater exposure to the risk of shotgun-carrying visitors than a suburban facility.

In a very real sense, the degree of risk facing health care facilities today is greater where managed care has made substantial inroads. Patients' natural anxieties may be boosted several notches by frustration when they are, for example, unable to gain authorization from their HMO for emergency care or for specific procedures they believe they need. They and their family and friends may feel thwarted by an ever-growing rank of restrictions, not all easy to understand, let alone to appreciate. Furthermore, cutbacks on every level of the health care delivery system are resulting in longer waits for care in many places, so that waiting rooms can turn into tinderboxes. As health care reform speeds up the rate of significant change, sometimes alarmingly so, security professionals need to stay on top of the emotional effects on patients, visitors, and staff.

For any health care facility, crimes and other serious incidents (such as fires) can be costly in terms of dollars and damage to the reputation of the organization. In addition to problems with employee morale and productivity as a result of security-related incidents, serious longer-term effects may be seen in staff recruitment and retention and in patient census.

■ *Taking Security Seriously*

How seriously a health care organization views its responsibility to provide a safe and secure environment can be seen by both the organizational and physical placement of the security operation. Security that reports at a low level and occupies space in a corner of the basement will have a tough time providing a successful protection program. As organizations flatten out in this era of downsizing, there is some tendency to push security farther down in the organizational hierarchy, usually leading to a loss of effectiveness; timely decisions and funding are reduced, and sooner or later everyone gets the message that security is not a priority.

On the other hand, the security department should not report to the chief executive officer or the chief operating officer. Although position nomenclature varies from organization to organization, the proper level for security reporting is the vice president level. Vice presidents of human resources or facilities management are good choices to be responsible for the security function.

Offices and other physical space occupied by security also speak to the value placed on this function by the organization. Size is not as important as location. Security should be in a highly visible and accessible location within the main facility—not in the basement or in a remote trailer. In some facilities, the security offices are located in the main lobby; the emergency department is also a good choice.

There is no question that health care facility security is taken seriously by many professional, regulatory, and quasi-regulatory entities with varying degrees of authority. Some impose requirements, some offer assistance in the form of guidelines or other resources, and some do both. For a comprehensive list, see Figure 1.3.

Knowing that actively promoting a safe and secure environment is a moral and legal necessity for every health care facility does not tell you what kind of security program is right for your particular facility. How big should it be? What should it do? The only way to answer these questions appropriately is to undertake a formal review of the basic risks inherent in the environment.

It is not true that all security incidents can be predicted or avoided. It is true that a sound protection program—custom tailored to fit the specific people, property, and circumstances found at your facility—will greatly lessen the impact of such an incident, as well as the odds of its occurring in the first place.

ORGANIZATIONS INVOLVED IN HEALTH CARE SECURITY

- **American College of Emergency Physicians**
  Publication: Emergency Department Violence: Prevention and Management.
  PO Box 619911, Dallas, TX 75261.

- **American Hospital Association**
  Ad hoc committee report, Hospital Security Issues: A CEO Briefing Report.
  Safety and security certificate program through the American Society of
  Healthcare Engineering (ASHE). One North Franklin, Chicago, IL 60606.

- **American Medical Association**
  Staff Report (B of T Report 23-I-94) referring to increased security in health
  care facilities with a focus on firearms in hospitals. 515 North State Street,
  Chicago, IL 60610.

- **American Society for Industrial Security**
  The largest security trade association in the world. Has a standing
  Healthcare Security Committee, newsletters, magazines, and educational
  seminars. 1655 North Fort Myer Drive, Suite 1200, Arlington, VA 22209.

- **Emergency Nurses Association**
  Resolutions concerning security in Emergency Departments and education
  programs. 230 East Ohio Street, #600, Chicago, IL 60611.

- **International Association for Healthcare Security and Safety**
  Established in 1968. The major trade association in health care security
  offering training programs, certification, certificates, educational seminars,
  newsletters, survey data, and journals. PO Box 637, Lombard, IL 60148.

- **Joint Commission on Accreditation of Healthcare Organizations**
  Security standards pertaining to accreditation and educational material and
  programs. One Renaissance Boulevard, Oakbrook Terrace, IL 60181.

- **National Center for Missing & Exploited Children**
  Educational programs, site inspections, and investigative support regarding
  infant abductions. Publication For Healthcare Professionals: Guidelines on
  Preventing Abductions. 2101 Wilson Boulevard, Suite 550, Arlington, VA
  22201.

- **Occupational Safety and Health Administration**
  Federal regulations and guidelines on protection requirements in the health
  care environment. U.S. Department of Labor, OSHA Publications, PO Box
  37535, Washington, DC 20213–7535.

Figure 1.3.   *These major organizations offer support for security programs
through books, magazines, seminars, and other educational tools.*

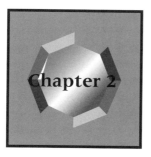

Chapter 2

Assessing Security Risks

The heart of the security management plan involves applying various safeguards to each security risk. A specified outcome for each safeguard then becomes an operating performance standard, as required by the Joint Commission.

The plan can be constructed by (a) first identifying risks and then determining the appropriate safeguard for each, which is the most common approach; or (b) by deciding first which safeguards will be used and then determining where each should be applied to the entire list of risks. The choice involves deciding between, for example, separately evaluating every location where the cashier function takes place and deciding how to handle them, one by one, and choosing to use closed-circuit television (CCTV) to manage a multitude of risks such as theft, trespass, and fire. The end result in both cases might be the use of CCTV to guard against theft at cashier stations, but the routes taken to arrive at this decision would differ.

Quantifying Risks

Either way it is approached, the objective of the risk assessment is to examine each and every function and physical space that make up the organization thoroughly to identify and quantify its individual security risk. The key question is: To what extent does a particular risk (theft, for example) in a particular function or area (say, neonatal care) pose a real or potential threat to the mission of the organization?

For this purpose, the facility is considered not as a single entity but as a group of discrete subenvironments—an animal research laboratory, a children's day care center, a restaurant, even a branch banking function. To each, the same complete set of security risks should be applied, from simple assault to civil disturbances and terrorism. (See Figure 2.1.)

In general, each risk will apply to each area to some degree, but the need to implement security measures to counter that risk will vary greatly. For example, the medical records function would be at high risk for the loss of information compared with the food service function; the food service is vulnerable to this loss to a lesser degree in the sense that (a) it is less likely to occur and (b) the consequences if it does occur are less severe.

There are two basic approaches to quantifying a risk. One is to assign the risk factor without regard to the security safeguards already in place and then to modify the factor by adding such protective elements. The risk of a fire in the loading dock, say, would be assigned a general factor based on the quality of its construction, its distance from the fire department, the presence of hazardous or highly flammable materials, (such as paint, fuels, and laboratory agents), and the proximity of heat sources. The next step would be to reduce the inherent risk involved, perhaps by installing sprinklers and fire extinguishers, instituting fire patrols, and training staff.

The second, more common approach, is to assign a risk factor that takes into account the safeguards already in place and the degree to which these are functioning properly. So that (to go back to our earlier example) the existence of a closed circuit television camera may lower the risk factor assigned to robbery of a

HEALTH CARE SECURITY RISKS

Personal	Property
Assault	Burglary
Simple	Gambling
Aggravated	Kickbacks/Fraud
Disturbances	Loss of information
Internal	Theft
External	Patient
Drug abuse	Staff
Homicides	Hospital
Hostage taking	Personal and property
Imposters	Civil disturbances
Kidnapping	Strikes
Robbery	Terrorism
Armed	Fire/Explosion
Unarmed	Bomb threats
Stalking	

Figure 2.1. *The same risks apply to a different degree in different areas of the hospital so that, for example, an animal research lab is much more vulnerable to bombing than a cafeteria.*

cashier station, but that factor would also need to reflect such real-world conditions as improper placement, inappropriate monitoring schedules, poor picture quality, or the lack of a backup video recording system.

Determining what security safeguards need to be improved or added to achieve an acceptable level of risk is a design rather than an assessment task, which will be taken up in Part II. The same is true of establishing an acceptable threshold or risk tolerance level. Some degree of risk will always be present, and each organization must determine, within the context of its own philosophy, what is and is not acceptable.

■ *Methodology*

Conducting a site-specific security assessment involves a review of data and reports, a review of staff input, and a hands-on inspection of the physical property.

The most commonly used documents are security incident reports for the past three to five years, safety committee records or reports, and area police statistics, which are a good indicator of the level of crime and crime trends in the neighborhood and which often provide valuable planning information.

Input from staff provides more specific information about security risks within a certain function or area. Someone who works in a given environment day in and day out will certainly have knowledge valuable to the security risk assessment, such as where and how money may be stored, the fact that a safe combination may not have been changed for years, and, most important, his or her own feeling of safety.

Those performing the assessment must be sensitive to perceived as well as real threats expressed by staff. A perceived threat that turns out not to be well founded may have little impact on the assessment of a risk but must be considered in the security plan design. An example might be employees who feel unsafe in a particular parking area, which a security review reveals to be properly protected with few or no incidents in the past record. The solution to these employees' misplaced concern may be as simple as providing them with information about the real situation. It may also require adding extra security to the lot, such as increased lighting, signage, or an emergency call system. Maintaining the perception of a safe environment among both staff and the public is an important objective of the security program.

The physical inspection must take into account the entire 24-hour operating period, as each hour may present different factors for review and evaluation. During the day, for example, access control to the materials management general store room would consist of department personnel, aided perhaps by card access, digital, or remote electrical lock release systems. This may be adequate protection against a break-in as long as the storeroom is occupied; however, illegal entry to this room may be a high risk at 3 AM or during the weekend. Night and/or weekend staff would undoubtedly provide input different than staff working Monday through Friday during the day.

Who Should Perform the Assessment? The assessment can be performed by anyone who possesses good management skills, a general business aptitude, and some health care security expertise. If an organization does not have access to someone with extensive experience in security they should do a comprehensive literature review in preparation. The medical center library staff would be helpful in identifying resource material, as would the International Association for Healthcare Security and Safety and the American Society for Industrial Security. (See Figure 1.3.)

It is common practice for health care organizations to hire an outside consultant to conduct the risk assessment and/or to design the security program to deal properly with the risks identified. It is important that such a consultant also have experience with security in the health care setting. He or she should be a certified health care protection administrator (CHPA, conferred by the International Association for Healthcare Security and Safety) or a Certified Protection Professional (CPP, conferred by the American Society for Industrial Security).

The facility security manager, director of facilities, and risk manager all are good candidates for conducting the security risk assessment. Although an assessment performed by an in-house staff member may lack objectivity, there are ways to compensate for this weakness; one is to use a team approach, another is to enlist the aid of a health care security manager from another organization in the community.

■ *Formats Vary*

There is no one right way to gather and record information during a security risk assessment. What is important is that the method used to facilitate a quantitative analysis results in a rating of the risks for each specific area or functional activity. A cross-reference format is often used. In Figure 2.2, a rating scale of 0–10 has been used to quantify security risks from no risk (0) to a risk of the highest degree (10). A rating of 5 or higher suggests that additional safeguards are required; a rating of 4 or lower indicates the risk is being properly managed.

"Properly managed" does not mean the risk has been eliminated, but that the probability of an incident has been reduced to a practical and realistic level. For example, the main cashier area may receive a risk rating of six relative to the exposure to armed robbery. The installation of a bullet-resistant glass across the service counter could bring that rating down to a three or lower. A multitude of security safeguards can be applied to a security risk to reduce the vulnerability. Figure 2.3 lists basic security safeguards that can be used in varying degrees or combinations to manage the security risk properly once that it has been identified and quantified.

Although each part of the facility must be reviewed separately, there will be some risks that also apply to the facility as a whole: fire, bomb threats, hostage taking, strikes, stalking. Still,

SAMPLE RISK ASSESSMENT WORKSHEET

Risks	Assault	Theft		Robbery	Drug abuse	Fire		
		Personal	Facility					
Area/Function								
Pharmacies								
Main	2	1	4	2				
6th Floor	2	1	3	2				
1250 Elm	4	3	3	8				
ED	6	2	3	7				
Nurseries								
Well baby	1	0	1	0				
Neonatal	1	0	1	0				
Sick baby	1	0	1	0				
Materials Management								
Main stores	1	1	6	1				
Dock	3	1	7	1				
Warehouse	2	1	5	0				
Medical Records								
Main	4	4	6	2				
Dead files	6	0	3	0				
Admitting	4	3	2	1				

Instructions: Each organization should add risks and areas/functions as appropriate. Place a number between zero (0) and ten (10) in each block to indicate the degree of security risk. A 0 indicates no risk and a 10 indicates a risk of the highest degree. Make 5 the cutoff level, so that a risk that rates a 5 or higher requires additional security safeguards to bring it down to an acceptable level of 4 or below. See Figure 2.3 for sample safeguards.

Figure 2.2. *Each organization will assess its various risks differently.*

BASIC SECURITY SAFEGUARDS

Security force

Staff security practices

Signage

Alarms—Panic and intrusion

Barriers—Walls, doors, glazing, fencing

Locking mechanisms

Lighting

Closed-circuit television

Identification of persons and property

Proper control procedures

Good hiring practices

Enforced security policies

Effective supervision of staff

Architectural traffic flow design

Secure containers storage (safes)

Landscaping (trimmed shrubbery and trees)

Figure 2.3. *Once security risk has been assessed, safeguards can be put in place to minimize that risk.*

these organization-wide risks are more likely to come into play in certain areas, and these should be specified as such. The risk of hostage taking, for example, would be greater in the emergency department or on a psychiatric unit than in the laundry or medical records department.

A major objective of the security risk assessment analysis is to identify security-sensitive areas, as the Joint Commission has specified. (See Figure 2.4.). Security-sensitive areas are those in which the mere existence of a specific function itself is a primary

COMMON SECURITY-SENSITIVE AREAS

Emergency department

Pharmacy

Medical records department

Mother/infant care

Cashier

General outpatient clinics

Specialized outpatient clinics (substance abuse, abortion)

Animal research laboratory

Mental health units

Figure 2.4. *Security-sensitive areas specific to an individual hospital might include a parking lot in a high-crime neighborhood.*

risk factor; these include birthing units, pharmacies, and emergency departments. Again, the size, scope, and exposure level of the function may mitigate the degree of actual risk. In terms of care of the newborn, for example, a nursery's vulnerability to a kidnapping would be greater in a large hospital than in a small six-bed maternity unit in a rural hospital.

Although some areas such as nurseries are considered to be security sensitive in all health care facilities, others are specific to hospitals, such as certain parking areas. Such parking areas would not pose a high risk by virtue of their function but because of their size, location, and exposure to repeated security problems.

In either case, the Joint Commission spells out specific requirements for safeguarding areas designated security sensitive in the Environment of Care standards.

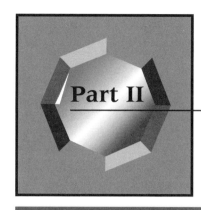

Part II

Security Plan
Basics

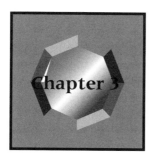

The Security Management Plan

The information gathered and analyzed in the security risk assessment guides the development of the security management plan. This is an outline of the organization's protection program, encompassing both the design and implementation of security safeguards.

Certain components of the plan, while not set in concrete, remain relatively constant, including statements of the security mission, the designated security responsibility, and the primary duties and responsibilities. Security operations, policies, and procedures, on the other hand, are subject to frequent change in response to information gleaned from the ongoing risk assessment process. (See Figure 3.1.)

Mission, Responsibility, Duty

The mission statement is the foundation of the security function. It spells out the reason the security department exists and its general approach to protecting the organization, and it does so in terms that relate to and support the broader mission of the organization itself. As long as it specifies the overall function and responsibility of the security program, the statement may take

BASIC COMPONENTS OF A SECURITY MANAGEMENT PLAN

Mission statement

Statement of assigned responsibility

Statement of primary duties and responsibilities

Vulnerability/risk assessment and evaluation

Sensitive-area designation and access controls

Security policies and procedures

Staff education and training

Security standards and performance measurements

Annual security evaluative report

Figure 3.1. *The security management plan serves as an outline for the entire security operation.*

any form considered appropriate, long or short; there is no set standard, format, or requirement. (See Figure 3.2.)

A specific person must assume responsibility for putting the mission statement into action—that is, for directing and managing the daily activities of the security department. The chief executive officer or chief operating officer of the organization must formally and in writing assign this security responsibility, generally designating a position—director of security, director of human resources, administrative vice president—rather than an individual.

The functions a security department performs vary widely within two primary categories: protection and service. The latter is easier to describe and to prescribe. A physician who locks himself or herself out of the office can readily see and, in fact, measure how long it takes security to respond and rectify the

SECURITY MISSION STATEMENTS: TWO EXAMPLES

1. The mission of the Department of Security is to protect and serve Memorial Hospital, patients, visitors, employees, medical staff, tenants, and all other persons on the hospital campus. We will accomplish this by the systematic and cost-effective integration of personnel, technology, and proactive and reactive programs.

   To carry out this mission, our primary areas of responsibility will include security, safety, fire protection, emergency preparedness and response, enforcement of laws and hospital regulations, and assistance to those in need.

2. United Hospital will exercise reasonable care in safeguarding patients and visitors, their property, the prevention of accidents, and the prevention of crime by taking appropriate action in times of emergencies. United Hospital will make every reasonable effort to comply with all appropriate health regulations, fire regulations, safety, and generally accepted security practices.

   Each department at United Hospital will formulate and publish safety and security rules and regulations that apply to activities of that department. Supervisors will instruct their employees in both general and specific safety and security practices. This training will be included as part of an initial orientation and through an ongoing in-service training process.

   Employees are expected to be aware of areas potentially hazardous to themselves, to patients, and to persons with whom they may come in contact. Employees are further expected to apply this knowledge in providing a safe, secure patient and work environment.

   The authority and responsibility for developing and implementing the general safety program rests with the Safety Committee as appointed by the chief executive officer. The chief executive officer will appoint a chairperson who will have the responsibility and authority as outlined by the Joint Commission on Accreditation of Healthcare Organizations.

Figure 3.2. *There is no one right way to compose a mission statement.*

situation. But the officer who is patrolling the physician office area and thereby diverts a thief is performing a function readily apparent to almost no one. This act of prevention, however—the crime that doesn't occur—is the essence of security.

During the last decade of organizational downsizing, security has been called upon—and, indeed, in an effort to justify program expenses, has offered—to provide more and more ancillary services. Inevitably, there is a gray area called "patient assistance" where service and protection come together and actually overlap.

One of the activities in this area is helping with combative patients, primarily in emergency departments, clinics, and psychiatric units. Do such patients pose a medical treatment problem or a security problem? Probably, the answer is both; a truly combative patient puts staff, and even visitors, at risk of assault. Security is more clearly the issue when medical staff merely suspect that a patient may become combative, or may decide to run away, and call on security to conduct a patient watch. It is not uncommon for security officers to spend up to 20% of their duty time in one form or another of patient assistance.

The potential conflict between proactive security protection and general services is highlighted in the following troubling example. A medium-sized hospital in a western state was staffed by two security officers around the clock. During the 11 PM staff shift change, one officer would patrol in the main employee/visitor parking lot and the second would patrol inside and outside the facility randomly. One evening, the officers, one right after the other, responded to "STAT" (emergency) calls from the emergency department (ED) to assist with two separate combative patients requiring restraints. Moments later, an employee arriving for work was abducted from the main parking lot, taken to a remote area off the property, and raped. In the lawsuit that followed, the employee plaintiff successfully argued that, having become accustomed to seeing an officer in the lot, she had an expectation of protection and that the officers were negligent in not providing it.

Had the first officer declined to respond to the ED call, claiming a duty to remain on proactive patrol in the parking lot—which had no previous history of security incidents, by the way—the physician or nurse in charge of the ED would most likely have had the security officer fired.

Might one officer have provided support for the ED while the other returned to normal duty? Possibly. But officers face the need to simultaneously perform more than one service or activity every day. Since it is impossible to spell out in advance which is the right decision in every situation (largely because not all situations are foreseeable), officers must act in accord with their own understanding of the priorities—which is why the mission statement is so important.

For a list of the many activities and services provided by today's health care security departments, see Figure 3.3.

Investigations

Which of these headlines is more likely to have resulted from an internal health care security investigation: "Pharmacist arrested on drug charges," or "Physician held on charges of molesting a patient." The answer is neither. A more realistic heading for a story on such an investigation—say, "Nurse fudges hours on time sheet"—is not going to sell many newspapers.

The fact is, while a criminal investigation or an arrest may follow from an internal security investigation, such outcomes generally are tangential to the purpose and scope of this kind of investigation. The vast majority of investigations required in the

SECURITY DUTIES, RESPONSIBILITIES, AND ACTIVITIES

Persons
Arrests
Assaults
Disorderly conduct
Door unlock
Drug impaired
Employee terminations
Escort
Forged/stolen prescription
Harassing communication
Illegal entry
Impersonation
Indecent acts/exposure
Larceny (personal)
Lifting help
Lost/missing keys
Misconduct
Missing patient
Obscene communications
Patient restraint
Possession of contraband
Property destruction and damage
Rape
Robbery
Safety breaches
Staff training
Suspicious person
Traffic accident
Trafficking
Trespass
Weapons

Injury/accident
Auto assistance
Directing traffic
Domestic conflict
Giving directions
Police assist
Regulating rules
Removing persons from property

Property
Arson
Facility lock/unlock
Found property
Gate controls
Larceny (facility)
Missing drugs
Missing property
Money escorts
Parking violations
Securing area
Towing vehicles

General
Alarm response
Alarm testing
Bomb threats
Courier runs
Disaster response
Fire response
Helicopter assist
Investigations
Raise/lower flag

The basis for this listing of typical duties and activities was furnished by the Security Department, Charlotte Mecklenburg Hospital Authority, Charlotte, NC.

Figure 3.3.   *Today's health care security department provides a variety of services and performs numerous activities.*

medical care facility are either noncriminal in nature or of such minor criminal status that they should not and do not receive any attention from a law enforcement agency.

A typical noncriminal security investigation involves alleged violations of policy, a fall down the front steps, false time recording, misuse of equipment or supplies, claims for damages, background checks, or sexual comments made by an employee. In the petty crime category are shoes missing from an employee locker, money missing from a patient's bedside table, an intentional scratch on a parked vehicle, and a missing bottle of a nonprescription drug. These may not warrant the attention of law enforcement, but left unchecked, they can result in a significant cumulative cost and a general escalation of minor law-breaking.

Another major type of security investigation is the examination of a situation to determine if, in fact, a crime or major loss has taken place. In one case, a general storeroom supervisor reported the theft of more than $22,000 worth of bedsheets and towels; the security investigation traced the loss to a bookkeeping error. Another common occurrence is the missing piece of office equipment, which turns out to have been not stolen but borrowed by another department or an employee taking it for home use.

The security investigation has at least two other very important objectives. One is deterrence: to serve notice that the organization does not tolerate wrongdoing and that even petty crime will be investigated. Second is to determine what steps and safeguards might be put into place to prevent a repeat of the incident.

The need for good, thorough security investigations should not be taken lightly by the organization. Performed discreetly and with respect for confidentiality, they may not be dramatic, but they yield a very high return on their investment.

■ *Records, Standards, Policies, and Procedures*

Records and reports—maintaining essential ones and eliminating superfluous ones—are important for security. (See Figure 3.4.) Since prevention itself cannot be accurately measured, many an insecure security department has compensated by setting up massive recording systems to document every single activity and service it performs, spending endless hours trying to show just how busy its officers are. In these archaic systems, one can find irrefutable evidence of how many times they answered the telephone, how many ID card pictures they took, how many night visitors they signed in, how many employees they escorted, how many parking notices they issued, ad nauseam. It is information no one needs to know.

ESSENTIAL SECURITY RECORDS AND REPORTS

Security incident reports

Security condition reports

Security officer daily activity reports

Measurement of security performance standards

Security incident/trending reports for review committee

Operational records (that is, lost and found, parking, investigations)

Administrative records (that is, time keeping, job descriptions, officer evaluations, training records)

Evaluation, feasibility, and planning reports

Annual security vulnerability and program review report

Figure 3.4. *Together, these records and reports provide a detailed picture of the security operation.*

If security incident reports and other essential record keeping is the lifeblood of the security program, standards, policies, and procedures constitute its backbone.

Performance Standards.   Performance standards, as required by the Joint Commission, can and should address both broad objectives (preventing crime) and specific outcomes (establishing the security response time to critical incidents). Another name for setting performance standards is benchmarking: giving the department a mark against which to measure itself, a way to know when it is performing satisfactorily.

Take the theft of patient property, which is always a basic security concern even when the actual dollar value of the property is not high. A standard regarding this crime might say that "every patient admitted to the hospital is informed of its policy regarding the amount of personal property patients may keep with them."

Performance Measurements.   In order to determine if a security performance standard is being achieved, it must be measured. In the standard cited above, a periodic audit or a sample patient population survey would determine if each patient had, in fact, been informed of the personal-property policy upon admission. When a standard is consistently not met, corrective action is required: reassessing the process, upgrading staff education, and, in extreme cases, imposing disciplinary measures.

Here are some samples of typical security performance standards and measurements:

Standard: All security intrusions and panic alarm systems will be 100% operational and function as intended.

Performance Measurement: All intrusion and panic alarm systems will be field tested (activated) the first week of each month; a report will be prepared and submitted to the director of security for an action required.

Standard: The security department will maintain a five-year file of adequately prepared security incident reports concerning facility security incidents; these will be filed chronologically by calendar year.

Performance Measurement: The facility security manager (or, in his absence, a designee) will review all security incidents prepared by security personnel daily except weekends and holidays. The director of security will randomly spot-check at least ten reports the first week of each month to evaluate the effectiveness of this standard and take any actions that may be required.

Standard: The security unit will maintain a security officer training level as follows: 50% International Association for Healthcare Security and Safety (IAHSS) or Certified Protection Officer (CPO) basic training certified officers; 100% IAHSS supervisory training certified supervisors (within three months of a person being hired or promoted to a security supervisory position).

Performance Measurement: A review of all security personnel training records will be conducted in the first week of January and the first week of July to determine compliance; a report will be prepared and submitted to the director of security for any action required.

Standard: The security department will respond to critical incidents with a high level of action to ensure a successful outcome.

Performance Measurement: Within 72 hours following a critical incident in which security participated (responded), there will be a debriefing meeting of the key people involved to review actions and to determine any modifications to the plan or further training that may be required.

When performance falls short of the standard, a thorough reassessment is required to determine what is at fault. Is the standard unrealistic? Is the system or the equipment faulty? Is officer training inadequate? One or more elements must be redesigned at this point.

Security Policies and Procedures.   Security policies and procedures—policies saying what must be done and procedures saying how—collectively can be thought of as an instructor's manual for the security department. Certain security policies are essential to all health care organizations—say, lock and key control—while others, such as policies concerning security for an animal research function, will be unique to the specific facility. (See Figure 3.5.) There should be policies to cover all conceivable security situations, no matter how unlikely some of these, such as hostage taking, may seem.

In many cases—fire safety, for example—security procedure will reflect the fact that the department has shared responsibility for implementing an organizationwide fire safety policy. On the other hand, policy and procedures concerning firearms on the premises probably will be the sole responsibility of security.

BASIC SECURITY POLICIES AND PROCEDURES

- Security staffing and deployment
- Facility access control
- Physical security system
- Documentation and records
- Training and education

  Security staff

  General staff
- Sensitive-area policy and procedure
- Area- and function-specific policies and procedures*

  VIP security

  Civil disturbance

  Patient assistance

  Lost and found

  Investigations

  Alarm monitoring and response

  Patient restraints

  Infant abduction response

  Helicopter landing support

  Visitor control

*Every organization will have specific security policies relative to its type of facility, mission, and environment. For example, a facility providing an employee day care center will specify security policies and procedures not needed or applicable to a facility that does not provide this service.

Figure 3.5. *Together, policies and procedures constitute an instruction manual for the security department.*

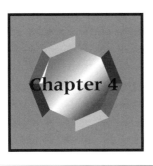

Chapter 4

Security
Staffing

The security department in a health care organization may use in-house employees (proprietary model), contractual employees (outsourcing), off-duty law enforcement officers, or a combination of these. (See Figure 4.1.) Regardless of which option it chooses, the organization is responsible for providing direction, control, and administrative support for the program, which includes the proper staffing, training, and equipping of security personnel.

■ Selecting the Staffing Model

Each staffing model has its strong and weak points. (See Figure 4.2.) The majority of health care organizations today have followed the lead of other major businesses in adopting the contract approach to security staffing. Although this trend is probably irreversible and certainly not incompatible with quality programming, hospitals too often use outsourcing solely to save money rather than to enhance the security function. The reality is that proprietary programs have generally become too expensive to operate.

A combination model, in which a proprietary program supplements in-house staff with contract personnel, may work in

SECURITY DEPARTMENT STAFFING MODELS

Proprietary (in-house)

Outsourcing (contract services)

Combination of proprietary and outsourcing

Law enforcement police

Combination of proprietary, outsourcing, and police

Figure 4.1. *Combination models can be the most difficult types of security staffing to implement.*

the short term but will most likely not survive as an effective staffing model, given the intense "we/they" feeling it tends to generate; in-house staff typically consider contract staff to be less qualified, often placing them in less desirable duty assignments, such as parking lot surveillance.

Even more problematic is the program staffed primarily by off-duty police or by in-house employees who have a dual responsibility for maintenance and security. The latter are clearly not going to be sufficiently focused on either aspect of the job, and the former are unlikely to be able to shift gears fast enough. Each organization must choose the model that works best for its unique situation.

■ *Selecting the Security Staff*

Once a model has been selected, the next step is to select the security personnel. The position description for each job category must set specific criteria in terms of both job function and qualifications. This includes physical requirements, which should be

CHARACTERISTICS OF SECURITY STAFFING MODELS

Type Characteristics	In-house	Contract	Combination	Off-Duty Police
Cost	High	Low/fixed	Moderate	High
Turnover	Low	High	Moderate	Moderate
Clear chain of command	Best	Good	Fair	Poor
Organizational control	Good	Best	Good	Poor
Effecting program change	Good	Best	Good	Poor
Upward mobility (career)	Fair	Good	Fair	N/A
Integration into organization	Best	Good	Good	Poor
Cost control	Poor	Best	Good	Poor
Health care expertise	Best	Fair	Fair	Poor
Supervision	Best	Good	Good	Poor
Training	Good	Fair	Fair	Poor

Figure 4.2. *These are subjective, rather than objective, judgments, based on the author's experience; other security experts might characterize these models somewhat differently.*

outlined in accordance with the Americans with Disabilities Act (ADA).

The same job description is used whether the personnel are in-house or contractual employees; if they are the latter, job qualifications should be included, along with wages and benefits, in the request for proposals from security companies and in the contract. The wages paid will have a direct bearing on the quality of personnel, but outsourcing is no reason to lower personnel standards.

Only rarely is the young security officer in it for the long haul. Security is simply not considered a primary career, except in the case of individuals who have prepared themselves academically and set out deliberately to gain experience that will lead them into security management. More often security becomes a second career for middle-aged persons who take early retirement or may for medical reasons be forced to leave another field.

A good candidate for a health care security officer position will not necessarily have had any background or experience in security. Often, previous experience in security or law enforcement actually necessitates more training, simply because there is so much to unlearn before such an individual is able to open his or her mind to the methods, procedures, and philosophy of health care security.

A good example of this problem can be seen in this case of a stolen gun. The gun was taken from an employee's car while it was parked in the hospital lot and the theft reported to the local police agency. But one of the hospital security officers on duty at the time of the incident, who was formerly with the police, couldn't let go of the case. Concerned that the gun could be used in a serious crime on the street, he was still investigating its disappearance some days later, neglecting to deal with several instances of theft involving patient and hospital property which he considered less important. His concern was not misplaced, simply misprioritized: Hired by the hospital to provide a secure environment for its staff, patients, and visitors, he was continuing to think and act first like a police officer, to whom a patient's missing watch, for example, would naturally take second place to a missing gun.

In addition to an open mind, basic traits common to good health care security officers include good verbal communication skills, a professional appearance and grooming, interest in helping others (compassion), common sense, and a high degree of integrity.

Although the selection and hiring process varies greatly from organization to organization, the background investigation of each candidate should include, at a minimum, the following:

Verification of activity and employment for the previous five years;

Check for criminal history;

A medical examination, including drug testing and other tests required by OSHA (the Occupational Safety and Health Administration);

A credit history; and

Feedback from previous supervisors and/or colleagues.

Equipping the Security Officer

The proper attire for security personnel has been the subject of considerable discussion. There are basically three options: a standard officer uniform, a blazer/slacks uniform, or regular street clothes (plain clothes). Street clothes are worn almost exclusively by security management personnel.

The standard officer uniform is used by the majority of field security officers, primarily for its effectiveness in deterring crime, projecting a feeling of security and safety, and attracting the attention of persons seeking assistance. In some programs, a standard uniform is used to identify field officers, while a blazer and slacks are worn by security supervisors and personnel primarily

engaged in providing directions or assistance, such as a reception-
ist or lobby attendant. The important thing about a blazer is that
its design should clearly say "security"—"unarmed security," that
is—to even the casual observer. Firearms should never be carried
by officers in blazers, even if they personally are authorized to
carry concealed weapons.

The number of armed security personnel in health care settings continues to decline each year, at least in part because of
the need for additional training and other associated costs, but
the debate over handguns for uniformed security personnel continues. (See Figure 4.3.) Among those convinced that the very
presence of a firearm can turn a dangerous situation into a
deadly one is the unarmed officer at a midwestern hospital who
was dispatched late one evening to investigate sounds coming
from the roof. Passing in front of a large air filter unit, the officer
was suddenly jumped from behind. After knocking the officer
down, the assailant waved his gun threateningly and fled down a
stairwell. This officer later remarked had he himself been armed,
his attacker would likely have felt compelled to shoot.

ADVANTAGES AND DISADVANTAGES OF ARMING THE SECURITY OFFICER	
Advantages	*Disadvantages*
Greater officer safety	Increased cost
Crime deterrent value	Training requirements
Increased staff feeling of safety	Greater liability

Figure 4.3. *Each hospital must decide for itself whether to arm some, all, or none of its security personnel.*

In any case, the most important piece of equipment the field security officer will carry is not a gun but a two-way radio, essential both for efficient response and for the safety of the officer. In the very small security operation, the cellular telephone may sometimes substitute for the radio. In general, the pager has limited use in security field operations.

In addition to the two-way radio, a field officer must be equipped with a flashlight, handcuffs, rubber gloves, notebook, and pen. (See Figure 4.4.) Other items are considered optional—as long as they don't add up to the appearance of someone who is ready to enter into battle with a fully loaded equipment belt.

■ *Size and Deployment of Security Staff*

The number of security personnel required to protect a specific campus properly cannot be derived from any specific formula. It depends on a number of factors, including the environmental setting, type and size of facility, programmed workload, number of requests for the routine or emergency services (called-for

---

BASIC ITEMS OF EQUIPMENT FOR THE SECURITY OFFICER

Two-way radio

Handcuffs

Flashlight

Baton (regular or collapsible)

Pepper spray

Rubber gloves

Notebook and pen

Figure 4.4. *The most important item on this list is the first.*

services), level of crime in the area, demographics, and acuity of care provided, as well as the level of security and service intended by the organization—that is, its true level of commitment, as expressed in funding and administrative support.

For example, a 200-bed medical care facility in a low-crime area with a low volume of activity might have one officer on duty around the clock (4.3 FTE). A facility of the same size in a high-crime area, with a broad scope of high-volume activity, might have a security staff of five to six officers on each shift, around the clock (25.8 FTE).

The terms *programmed workload* and *called-for service* require a closer look. The first refers primarily to activities that can be predicted and, in many cases, actually scheduled, such as the timed locking and unlocking of specified facility access points, including parking areas. Other examples of programmed workload are lost-and-found processing, in-service training and education of staff, required documentation, operating a shuttle bus, bank runs and other errands, relief for a telephone operator or other service personnel, formal fire extinguisher inspections, and the staffing of specific security posts.

The term *called-for service* refers to the demand aspects of the security workload, which are by nature somewhat unpredictable. These fall into two categories: demand calls for routine services, which can be anticipated to some extent, and demand calls for emergency services, which cannot. Calls for employee security escorts to and from parking areas, for example, are to be expected, while emergency (STAT) calls to deal with out-of-control patients generally come out of the blue; such calls most often come from the emergency department, psychiatric unit, or clinic setting but can originate at any place and time. In a recent case in Florida, two nurses were severely beaten by a patient on a hospice unit of the facility, resulting in hospitalization and a lengthy recuperation period for both.

One way to arrive at the appropriate-sized security department for a particular facility is to calculate the number of officers
required for the department to respond to emergency calls within
four minutes, which should be the performance standard.

More important than numbers to the level of security being
provided is staff deployment. Duty assignments are of two types:
fixed post or roving patrol. A fixed-post assignment does not necessarily mean a person is tied to a desk or simply stands in one
location. In the emergency department, for example, a fixed-post
assignment may call for an officer to move about the department
or a defined area within or around it. On the other hand, a night
entry access control point may require the officer to remain at a
specific location and be relieved by another officer for breaks. A
roving officer would normally be assigned a geographical area,
where he or she would provide a preventive patrol function and
be available to respond to service requests.

It is common for an individual's duty shift to include both
fixed post and roving assignments. An officer working a 4 PM to
midnight shift, for example, might be scheduled as follows:
Patrol, provide relief for a dispatcher, patrol, then assume a fixed
post in a parking area during a shift change. Depending on the
structure of the program, this officer may or may not be permitted to abandon the fixed post to answer a call.

A major objective in designing officer deployment schedules
is high visibility, which, again, provides both a deterrent effect
and a feeling of security. The end of visiting hours in the evening
or a staff shift change is no time for officers to be patrolling
closed areas or writing a report in the security office. One means
of achieving this high level of visibility is to overlap security shifts
during peak periods—that is, start a new shift an hour or two
before the old one ends. A hospital that normally deploys one
officer around the clock, for example, might start the normal
midnight shift at 10 PM so that two officers would be present

during this busy period; with this schedule, seven ten-hour shifts for the week will result in coverage 26 hours consecutively. In some cases, part-time personnel can be used for double or triple coverage during key time periods.

Another method of achieving high visibility is to keep officers out of the security office—particularly when that office is (misguidedly) located in a remote spot. A partial solution to this problem is to create special report-writing areas in high-traffic locations, such as in the main lobby, clinic waiting rooms, or the waiting area of the emergency department. Most of these sites offer a counter or desk that officers can use; if not, a small writing desk can be placed in a corner. Not only are the officers readily identifiable and available to persons seeking assistance, but they generally find they need less time to prepare reports!

■ *Security Officer Training*

Training is one of the most important aspects of a good protection program. To some people, training means basic preparation to successfully complete everyday tasks. To others, it implies a more advanced skill level that extends to the proper handling of extreme emergencies; certainly, there should always be at least one security officer trained to this level. In any case, training is literally a never-ending task, required throughout the employment period of every officer. (See Figure 4.5.)

Basic preassignment training is short-term classroom instruction in the elements of security service as applied to the health care environment. This segment of training, which typically requires six to eight hours of classroom time, includes education about blood-borne pathogens and general safety, as required by OSHA. (See Figure 4.6.)

Pre/postassignment training is often referred to as on-the-job training (OJT). During this time, the officer learns the specific

---

CATEGORIES OF SECURITY OFFICER TRAINING

Basic preassignment

On-the-job (pre, post)

Periodic in-service

Skills improvement

Basic certification (International Association for Healthcare Security and Safety)

Special certification (cardiopulmonary resuscitation)

Professional development

Figure 4.5. *Training is an ongoing process, tailored to the needs of both new officers and veterans.*

tasks to be performed for each duty shift, and reviews general security duties and responsibilities. How long this takes depends on the complexity of the assignments and the learning curve exhibited by the trainee, but it is generally between 10 and 40 hours. Officers should not be permitted to fill a regular duty post until OJT training has been successfully completed, as indicated on an OJT checklist. (See Figure 4.7.) This checklist should be signed by both the trainee and the trainer, who may be the facility security manager, a shift supervisor, or a regular shift officer who has been designated the training officer. Trainees often wear street clothes or a special training uniform. This practice heads off the perception that officers are doubling up or being used to perform services for which they are not properly trained.

Periodic in-service training usually is provided monthly or quarterly in the form of demonstrations, classroom instruction, video presentations, and guest speakers from within and outside the organization. A yearly training calendar should be prepared to

TYPICAL PREASSIGNMENT TRAINING TOPICS

The role of the health care security officer

Security department organizational structure

Customer/public relations

Patrol techniques and procedures

Critical incident response procedures

Fire prevention and control

Report preparation and utilization

Use of basic equipment (radio)

Basic safety

Preliminary investigation procedures

Figure 4.6.   *Many of these topics may be addressed again in refresher courses or from a different perspective in more advanced training.*

indicate subject matter, dates, and locations. Often these programs serve as refresher courses on subjects such as emergency response procedures, de-escalation techniques, and customer service. Between 18 and 32 hours are devoted to this segment of training each year; usually all shifts attend programs together, but shorter presentations may be given on each shift.

Skills training is provided for discrete tasks or functions, such as weapons use, cardiopulmonary resuscitation, and computer processing, specific to the individual facility security program. The subject matter, duration, and other aspects of such training often are mandated by law or other guidelines.

The International Association for Healthcare Security and Safety (IAHSS) provides two types of training programs. The first is a certification program for basic officer training that meets the basic training standard first adopted by IAHSS in 1975; a revised 1995 *Basic Training Manual and Study Guide* is available from the

SAMPLE ON-THE-JOB TRAINING (OJT) CHECKLIST

(OJT) CHECK SHEET

Employee's Name   Facility

Orientation and OJT are very important components of an overall training program. In order to assure that the vital components of a security/parking officer's position are adequately conveyed and adequately understood, the following checklist is to be used for documentation purposes.

Please verify the training for each item is covered. The trainer, as well as the trainee, shall initial next to each item. Upon completion of the entire check sheet it shall be forwarded to the corporate office for inclusion in the employee's record.

Area of Training	Initials Trainee	Initials Trainer	Date
Introduction with facility supervisor.			
Familiarization with campus ground and buildings (will receive a map).			
Review-understanding of DARs and facility orders.			
Fire response—alarm procedures—fire panel, hydrant, and building sprinkler system standpipe locations.			
Familiarization with building locks/keys.			
Review of campus interior, and exterior disaster plans.			
Department support—checks and location of mechanical rooms, boiler room, and research.			
Introduction with shift boiler operator.			
Introduction with facility manager.			

Note: Initials indicate the trainee has received and understands the above listed training. Trainer initials indicate the appropriate information has been conveyed to the best of the trainer's ability.

Supervisor's Name	Date of completion/submission of forms

Figure 4.7.   *Each member of the security force must go through the same steps but at his or her own pace.*

association. (See Figure 4.8.) Students completing study of this manual and of the current Joint Commission security standards may apply to take the basic certification examination administered by the association by writing IAHSS, PO Box 637, Lombard,

---

INTERNATIONAL ASSOCIATION FOR HEALTHCARE SECURITY AND SAFETY (IAHSS) BASIC TRAINING STANDARD: UNITS OF INSTRUCTION

I. Introduction to Health Care Security
The health care organization
Security as a service organization
Public/community/customer relations
Employee/labor relations

II. Fundamental Security Skills
Patrol and post procedures/techniques
Security interaction with patients, visitors, and employees
Self-protection/self-defense
Professional conduct and self-development
Crisis intervention
Interview and investigation
Report preparation/writing
Report utilization
Judicial process/courtroom procedure/testimony

III. The Security Role in Health Care Operations
Nursing units
Business office
Pharmacy
Emergency and mental health units
Support units/auxiliary services

IV. Protective Measures
Health care vulnerabilities/risks
Access control concepts/systems
Physical security measures
Equipment usage/maintenance

V. Health Care Safety and Emergency Preparedness
Basic safety concepts
Fire prevention
Fire control response
Bomb threats/procedures
Disaster control/response
Civil disasters

VI. Security and the Law
Criminal and civil law
Narcotics and dangerous drugs
Public safety interactions/liaisons

Figure 4.8. *The International Association for Healthcare Security and Safety also offers supervisory and safety training.*

IL 60148. The second type of association program offers certificates for supervisory training and for safety training for the health care security officer.

Staff development is a combination of training and education, offered in fulfillment of the organization's duty to foster and provide the opportunity for self-development. This may mean more in-depth education in security subjects or on general health care principles. Preparation for advancement may include supervisory training, as well as college courses.

An individual training record must be maintained for each security officer, documenting all training of every kind he or she receives while employed by the organization. In addition to being a standard of the IAHSS, this is simply good management. The association standard requires that security officers be given a copy of their training record upon leaving the organization.

Security Officer Competency

A training program is not complete unless the lessons learned have been successfully applied to everyday security operations. Can the officer assist, patrol, and inspect? Can he or she carry out assignments and respond to emergency situations in a professional and effective manner? Competency, the outcome of training, can be measured to some extent through exams and controlled demonstrations, but everyday job performance is the true test.

Quantifying the level of a security officer's performance is a cyclical process, which uses many different methods in addition to the time-honored pencil-and-paper test. These include supervisory surveillance and dialogue, formal evaluations, critique of incidents, review of reports, and customer feedback. When and where deficiencies are identified, training or retraining should follow, unless a determination is made that an officer simply is not a candidate for continued employment.

Ongoing documentation of the officer's progression through the training process is an essential part of program administration. It allows measurement of the performance of the indivdual and the department: This is the level we must attain, this is the best we can do, this is the record we must beat.

■ *The Critical Incident*

The most dramatic test of an officer's training may be a radio message: "Security—respond to a shooting in the Pavilion II Clinic." Although most security officer training is geared toward the routine tasks associated with health care security, one day— any day, anywhere in the facility—a critical incident will take place: an event out of the ordinary that endangers lives or property and requires immediate action to reduce or contain the risk. (See Figure 4.9.)

It might be a fire, a civil disturbance, or a natural disaster— three examples of critical incidents for which there should be specific action plans in place. It may be a large water leak, an electrical outage, or a hazardous material spill, none of which are, strictly speaking, security incidents but which security personnel may be expected to help resolve.

Whether it comes in the form of an intrusion or panic alarm, a disruptive patient, a fire, or a major criminal act, the critical incident is the ultimate test of individual officers and the department as a whole. Until it passes this test, the security function is, in essence, on probation.

CRITICAL INCIDENT RESPONSE GUIDELINES

Proceed quickly and safely to the scene. Never run to the scene; observers may become frightened unnecessarily. Arrive in a composed manner. Survey the scene before cautiously proceeding into the area.

Obtain basic information. Gather facts about who, what, when, where, and how. Evaluate the nature and extent of the problem to determine an initial course of action.

Alert others when appropriate. Timely communication of pertinent facts can greatly affect the outcome of events. Others to notify may include another security officer, a security supervisor, a hospital supervisor or administrator, the police or fire departments, and others potentially affected by the incident.

Direct actions at the scene. Never take action that unnecessarily endangers yourself or others. Injury to yourself or others and further damage may be avoided when proper leadership is exhibited. Once proper authorities have arrived, leadership should be turned over to them.

Secure the scene. Eliminating unnecessary observers, identifying witnesses, and preserving evidence improves the chances of a successful conclusion to the incident.

Complete required documentation. Take written notes and obtain verbal or written statements that may be used later in preparing a final report of the incident. Assist others in preparing documentation when appropriate.

Figure 4.9. *Guidelines like these enable officers to tackle even the most unfamiliar events calmly and confidently.*

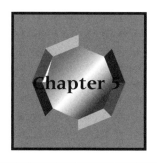

The Use of Physical Security

Integrated systems, open and closed architecture, and digital compression are just some of the buzzwords heard today in the world of electronic security. Electronic security is moving forward at a fast pace and already plays a significant role in creating effective security systems. Just as important, however, are the time-tested staples of physical security, which include lighting, fencing and other barriers, signage, glazing (glass and bullet-resistant acrylics), and, of course, the security officer—all essential elements in the arsenal of security safeguards.

Most physical security safeguards are designed to manage or control access, that is, to channel traffic in the manner desired and to deny or discourage intrusion by unauthorized persons into a specific area. Locks are intended to deny access; signs are intended to discourage it.

◼ Integrated Security Systems

Not that long ago, security programs commonly used various electronic security devices in a series of stand-alone systems. For example, there might have been an intrusion alarm system side by side with an item of closed-circuit television (CCTV) equipment, and next to that a small system that electronically operated a lock on a door or a receiving dock gate. In electronic terms, these individual systems did not talk to each other. They required numerous computers and other redundant equipment, to say nothing of excessive installation costs and space needs.

Enter the integrated systems approach. In simplistic terms, the idea is to use one computer (with a backup) to run the entire system, into which all equipment is consolidated. The security application for an emergency fire exit door is one example: When the door is opened, an alarm device is activated, triggering a CCTV camera to focus on the exit. As this occurs, the CCTV picture is brought up on a large screen, alerting the monitoring officer. At the same time, a videotape recorder is automatically activated. Because each of the devices is fully integrated with the others, all these events occur within a split second.

Now assume that the obstetricians need to be able to use this same door without the security devices going into alarm mode. It is a simple matter to install an electronic digital key pad, or electronic card reader, to operate the lock and shunt out the alarm device. It is now an alarmed exit door permitting authorized access. In this application, a shunting device would be required on each side of the door to allow both entry and exit for authorized persons.

■ *Closed-Circuit Television*

The use of CCTV in health care security has undergone great changes in recent years, caused in part by advancing technology and in part by changes in protection philosophy. Technologically, CCTV systems have become more affordable, more dependable, more innovative, and smaller. Cameras the size of a small matchbox deliver exceptional quality today, and CCTV color systems have become as affordable as black and white. One of the new applications of this latter development is the video identification system, in which a person's picture is stored on videotape for viewing at any time; it also can be transferred to an identification badge.

The transmission of CCTV signals has been a limiting factor in some security applications. The most commonly used signal transmission method has been the coaxial cable, which requires a direct connection between camera and monitor. Although microwave links and other transmission methods have been available for some time, their cost has made them prohibitive for most facilities. Now, new and upgraded methods of signal transmission are being introduced that will open up new security applications—and not a moment too soon, as mergers and affiliations are putting new and different demands on security communication systems for geographically widespread health care systems.

Centralized vs Noncentralized CCTV Applications.   Large CCTV security monitoring stations, with many banks of television monitors, are a thing of the past. Such systems used either one monitor for each camera or a sequential switcher, which would rotate images from one camera to another on a timed basis. Although this method reduced the number of monitors required, it obviously limited the views from any given camera to the time slot allowed by the rotation. Further, the protection afforded by this type of system was of questionable value, given the frailty of human nature: It is simply not possible for one individual to monitor a bank of video screens effectively for any significant time, as one security officer in a large medical center learned to her chagrin. It was only after her shift was over that she saw, on videotape, the assault that occurred in full view of a camera she was monitoring at the time. Although she swears she never dozed off, she nonetheless missed the full 12 seconds of critical action.

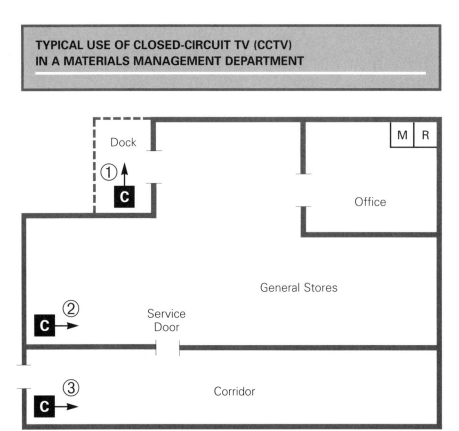

**TYPICAL USE OF CLOSED-CIRCUIT TV (CCTV)
IN A MATERIALS MANAGEMENT DEPARTMENT**

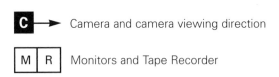

Camera and camera viewing direction

| M | R |
Monitors and Tape Recorder

Figure 5.1. *As used here, CCTV has surveillance, control, and deterrence value.*

Today's strategic security planning has led to widespread use of the decentralized, or departmental, approach to CCTV. Good examples of this application are often found in emergency departments, birthing units, pharmacies, and, as in Figure 5.1, materials management areas. In this figure, one person—the department secretary or clerk—can easily see all access areas at once. The primary safeguards are the receiving clerk and store-room personnel; however, as they move about doing their respective jobs, there is a loss of access control. The CCTV system provides extra surveillance and control of this vulnerable area and, with cameras in full view, adds the element of deterrence. Outsiders presumably do not know the capability (or limitations) of the system; they do not know where additional cameras may be, who may be watching, or if the system contains a tape recorder.

In any given security program there may be a mix of central-ized and decentralized applications of CCTV. A central security monitoring area may keep an electronic eye on areas that are not being viewed elsewhere, and provide redundant or backup view-ing of certain strategically placed, decentralized camera locations. For example, the materials management system shown in Figure 5.1 has a camera on the dock area. Because the department is closed during off-hours, this camera is also monitored in the cen-tral system, which provides redundant viewing during the regu-lar workday and then takes over at night.

There are at least two other good reasons for the decentral-ized use of CCTV. First, it is considerably cheaper than the cen-tralized approach. Second, it reminds personnel that the primary responsibility for security belongs to the individual department, with the security department providing additional resources and backup.

Basic CCTV Concepts for Security. A general rule for using CCTV for security purposes is that the system should be designed to videotape all events, or at least be capable of taping on demand at a system-generated signal. A camera set to view persons enter-ing or leaving a neonatal unit, for example, should be taping continuously. A camera fixed on an emergency fire exit need only tape as necessary, when someone moves into the field, at which point a motion sensor or similar device would automatically trigger the taping process. In a third scenario, a person monitoring general parking areas may manually activate a recorder at his or her discretion. There are videotape recorders to fit virtually every need, including those that record multiple cameras on a single videotape, those with various speed settings, and those that record the time and date directly onto the image.

How long should CCTV videotapes be retained? This varies with the application. A tape that records persons who are accessing a medicine storeroom may need to be kept longer than one recording vehicles that enter and exit a parking area.

In any CCTV security system, the objective and intended use of each camera should be written into the security operation plan, indicating the monitoring times and whether it is intended for general surveillance as a supplement to other safeguards or for direct control of a function or activity. In the case of the materials management CCTV in Figure 5.1, the security operations plan might read as follows:

> There are three CCTV cameras and one four quad monitor used in the access control function in the general storeroom and receiving dock area. This system is intended to supplement the access control effected by personnel working in the department; it is randomly monitored by the general stores clerk in the storeroom office from 8 AM to 5 PM, Monday through Friday. All cameras are tape recorded, with the tape changed each working day by the storeroom clerk. The tape will be held for three working days unless circumstances dictate holding it for longer.

> *Camera objectives:*

> *Camera #1* provides a general surveillance of loading, unloading, and temporary storage of materials on the receiving dock.

Camera #2 provides a view of persons entering the storeroom from the public corridor.

Camera #3 provides a view of persons exiting the storeroom, including materials being removed.

The use of fake or "dummy" CCTV cameras is almost always a bad idea in situations where it might imply that the system is providing an element of security and safety for individuals. In a gift shop, where everyone understands that it is meant to control shoplifting, this practice may be tolerated.

■ *Alarm Systems*

Cost effective, efficient, and reliable are all accurate descriptors of security alarm systems. The alarm is an essential element in the health care facility protection program regardless of the size of the organization.

Security alarms come in two types: the intrusion alarm and the panic (holdup/emergency) alarm. The term intrusion is often associated with a break-in; more broadly speaking, it means an invasion of space that may require an immediate response, simple surveillance, or the creation of a record that can be audited.

An alarm system is made up of three primary components: activation device, signal transmission, and enunciation (sounding system). Each component offers an array of options suitable for specific applications. Activation devices include manual push buttons, magnetic door contacts, motion/thermal sensors, and glass break sound detectors, to name just a few. Methods of signal transmission include hard wire, radio waves, microwave, fiber optic, and regular telephone lines. The enunciation of the signal can be in the form of bells, chimes, sirens, digital readouts, printouts, or any combination of these.

Although most alarm systems today are computerized and centrally monitored, there are still some door alarms that activate and sound only at the specific door point. This stand-alone type of alarm is generally a battery-operated, self-contained unit, of limited value in providing any real protection and often providing nothing but irritation instead. The alarm requires a great deal of maintenance, including battery replacement, and is often not heard by anyone—or else it is heard by everyone, interminably it seems, until someone arrives with a key to silence it.

Intrusion-Alarm Applications.   The fire emergency exit door and stairwell doors leading to or from critical areas such as psychiatry, surgery, or birthing units are common intrusion-alarm applications. Control devices allow authorized use of such doors while the alarm system offers basic protection. Other areas where intrusion alarms can be effective are in general storerooms, warehouses, gift shops, cashier and safe areas, medical records, pharmacies, and other critical locations not occupied by staff on a continuous basis.

Panic-Alarm Applications.   As workplace violence increases, so does the use of panic-alarm systems, meaning systems that signal when immediate security assistance is needed at a given alarm activation point. These include pharmacies, cashier stations, gift shops, and remote work areas. In the health care setting, the panic alarm is also widely used to request additional medical assistance, most often in emergency treatment rooms and on psychiatry units.

The most widely used panic alarm activation device is a button affixed to a wall or under a counter. Foot-activated devices, expensive and prone to fail, are rarely used; they are often right where a person would naturally want to rest his or her feet and, if moved out of the way, just as often end up being inaccessible in an emergency. Some systems on the market use a small activation device carried or worn by the individual. However, pinpointing the exact location of this person when he or she activates the device requires extensive and somewhat expensive installations.

Three fundamental concerns, or limitations, are connected with the panic-button alarm system. First, the person who activates the system has no way of knowing that the device is operating correctly and that the intended signal transmission has actually occurred. Second, it is too easy to activate the device accidentally. Third, some people find irresistible the temptation to conduct a personal test of the system, to see how long it takes for a response—something that should only be tested by authorized personnel under controlled circumstances.

■ *Computerized Access Control*

At Community Hospital, a new computer was delivered to the general storeroom Friday afternoon. It is now Monday morning and the shelf where it was placed is empty. Within three hours of the first report to security, the computer is recovered. "It was elementary," said a security staffer. There was no activation of the intrusion-alarm system over the weekend. There were, however, seven "card authorized entries," as documented in an access control system audit report produced by computer. Each person who accessed the storeroom apparently had a legitimate reason for doing so—except one. The exception was a new materials management employee, who, according to the audit report, entered at 3:30 PM Sunday afternoon, not realizing that the time and date of each card use was captured by a computer.

The security investigation revealed that the employee's access card, which should have allowed him entrance only during the regular Monday–Friday work shift, had inadvertently been programmed to allow 24-hour access. Had it been programmed correctly, the access card simply would not have worked that Sunday afternoon. (In fact, some systems will record attempts to use a card during unauthorized times.)

When used properly, such a computer access control system is the most cost-effective physical security element available. Access control systems come in all shapes and sizes and most price ranges. Once the functional (operational) security system has been designed, a security systems (engineering) consultant can help an organization settle on the most appropriate option.

One Card, Many Uses. The front-end cost of a computerized access control system is the biggest expense in a protection system. What makes the system cost effective is the multiple functions it can perform, the level of protection it can apply, the instant adjustments it can make spontaneously in security situations, and, most important, the money that is not spent trying to use old and outdated access control systems. A three-year return on investment is a realistic goal. This means that a million-dollar system, if properly designed and implemented, will have paid for itself in 36 months.

In a typical card access system, the card:

Serves as the staff identification badge;

Activates the parking gate;

Allows entry through the employee's locked entry point;

Records time for pay purposes;

Acts as a charge card at the cafeteria or pharmacy;

Controls the dispensing of scrubs and other materials, including drugs;

Allows entry into the locker room, lounge, or work area;

Serves as a facility library card; and

Allows entry into the medical record system.

A by-product of this multiple use concept is that there is a high degree of compliance with the requirement that persons wear the badge while on facility property. Even reluctant medical staff are willing to wear this identification badge when they understand its real value.

The increased level of protection afforded by the card access control system can be measured in a number of ways. The staff immediately *feels* more secure and, in fact, the number of strangers wandering about the facility is decreased dramatically. More tangibly, theft is reduced by as much as 50%, which by itself can return that $1 million investment to some organizations in record time.

An example of a system instantly adjusting spontaneously to a security situation involves the staff member who is terminated or arrested for assault against another staff member, in either case threatening to get even with the organization. A single stroke at the keyboard will invalidate the person's access card, rendering it useless. So although it is always important to retrieve the computerized card access identification badge at termination, thanks to this feature it is not as critical as retrieving keys or nonprogrammable access cards.

The computerized system saves a significant amount of money in hardware, labor, and supplies associated with traditional lock-and-key systems. Key accountability is not only costly, it defies the best of intentions to maintain system integrity. Replacement of the first missing key begins the integrity erosion process, to say nothing about the number of keys reproduced without authorization or accountability. Some systems offer control over the reproduction of keys but this feature is extremely expensive. And even if keys can be properly accounted for, there still is no way to be sure that a "legitimate key" has not been used "illegitimately" to enter a controlled area.

In short, although there will always be a use for traditional lock-and-key systems in the health care environment, they should be limited to areas and functions designated "low security priority," such as small storage areas, desks, cabinets, and some offices.

Computerized Access Control Technologies. In most computerized access control systems, a card is used to activate a reader. However, in addition to different card technologies, there also are biometric readers that read fingerprints, the eye, or the voice. (See Figure 5.2.)

The emerging technology of choice in health care security is the proximity card. The "prox" card, as it is commonly called, has several advantages over the other technologies, starting with the fact that it has no slot and, if desired, can be mounted in walls or

---

COMMON CARD-ACCESS TECHNOLOGIES

Bar code

Barium ferrite

Magnetic stripe

Proximity

Wiegand

Infrared

Figure 5.2. *The convenient proximity card is increasingly favored over other technologies.*

behind other barriers. This feature renders the system virtually vandal proof. There is little maintenance, since there are no components to get dirty or wear out. The greatest advantage however, is convenience: The prox card only needs to come within the "reading field" to activate the reader, which allows users a "hands-free read" with quick entry.

■ *Other Physical Security Devices*

The Combination Lock.   Electrical and mechanical combination locks are in fairly wide use today. The obvious advantages of this type of lock are (a) not having to issue and retrieve keys and (b) the fact that it is both easy and relatively cheap to change the combination. On the other hand, the combination is easily compromised by word of mouth, and getting a new one out to all those affected can be a major project. This type of lock should be considered a screening device, helpful where there are minimal security needs—locker areas, lounges, small storage areas—and a large number of users.

Glazing.   The term glazing refers to any transparent or translucent material used in windows, doors, or walls to admit light. Products range from common window glass to bullet-resistant acrylic materials, which are important for safety as well as security in that they prevent breakage and injury. Acrylics are most often used to protect service counter areas at cashier stations, admitting, triage areas, and pharmacy service windows. The cost of glazing is determined by the thickness of the material, which relates to the degree of protection required. Acrylics are generally more expensive to glaze than glass. Although very thin acrylic may provide sufficient protection, it usually will require more frame support than glass.

Signage.   Security signs are used to inform ("No Smoking"), deter ("All persons must pass through metal detector"), and dissuade people from engaging in certain behaviors ("Authorized Personnel Only"). (See Figure 5.3.) Signs are also helpful to security personnel who are responsible for confronting strangers and enforcing rules and regulations. An "Authorized Personnel Only" sign, for example, makes it easier to ask persons who are not displaying an identification badge to state their business—tactfully, of course.

One of the most important security signs does not look like one at all: the prominent sign indicating the night entrance for the public. In the very large facility there may be more than one such entrance; often the emergency department walk-in entrance doubles as a night entrance for both the public and employees.

Security Barriers.   Protective barriers include walls, doors, shrubs, fences, and natural land barriers. In exterior (grounds) applications, fencing, walls, and shrubs can be used indepen-

---

COMMON HEALTH CARE SECURITY SIGNS

Authorized Personnel Only

Not Responsible for Items Left in Change Rooms

Premises Being Monitored by Electronic Surveillance

Firearms Prohibited on This Property

All Lockers Subject to Inspection

All Persons Must Pass through Metal Detector

Door Alarmed

Figure 5.3.   *Signage lends authority to rules and regulations.*

dently or in combination with each other. Height generally indicates the degree of security intended: The four- or five-foot barrier is used to define property lines and to create desired traffic patterns, while barriers six to eight feet tall are used to deter entry or exit. Barbed wire topping is sometimes used to compensate for lack of height and to secure high-risk areas such as the central oxygen storage tank area. Shrubs, which cannot be climbed, or a thorny plant can enhance both the protective and the aesthetic environment.

Night Lighting and Foliage. On many health care campuses, a clear line of sight requires the proper pruning of foliage to eliminate hiding places and to obtain maximum benefit from night lighting, which is frequently a focus in premises liability litigation cases. Since trees often obstruct the light source, lighting inspections should obviously be conducted before the leaves fall in autumn or after they return in the spring.

There are commonly accepted night security lighting standards. (See Figure 5.4.) A burned-out lamp (bulb) does not necessarily mean that there is not a sufficient light source to meet the minimum standards, nor does it necessarily require immediate corrective action. It is quite common to use multiple light sources to achieve the desired light levels specifically to compensate for an individual malfunction. This makes it possible to batch the maintenance of night light sources mounted high on poles that, because they can only be serviced with a boom truck, would otherwise be cost prohibitive.

■ *Security through Environmental Design*

The layout and design of campus grounds, building exteriors, and internal building areas is yet another consideration in the achievement of cost-effective security. There is actually a formal

NIGHT SECURITY LIGHTING STANDARDS

Lighting standards are grouped into the following four zones:

Zone I

■ 2.0 foot candles (FC) for building entrances and exterior walls, to a minimum height of 8 feet, for vital locations or structures
■ 1.0 FC for roof surfaces requiring surveillance

Zone II

■ 1.0 FC for parking lots
■ 0.4 FC for roadways
■ 0.2 FC for storage areas
■ 0.2 FC for walkways

Zone III

■ 1.0 FC for parking lots
■ 0.4 FC for roadways
■ 0.2 FC for walkways
■ 0.1 FC for storage areas
■ 0.05 FC open areas

Zone IV

■ 2.0 FC for pedestrian entrances
■ 1.0 FC for roadway entrances
■ 1.0 FC for rail entrances
■ 0.2 FC on vertical plane, at points 3 feet above the ground, for "glare
  barrier"
■ 0.1 FC for fence line (nonisolated)
■ 0.05 FC for water approaches
■ 0.05 FC for open areas
■ 0.05 FC for boundary line (isolated fence or no fence)

Source: Based on *IES Lighting Handbook* 5th ed, New York: Illuminating Engineering Society, and
American National Standard Practice for Protective Lighting, New York: Illuminating Engineering Society
(345 East 47th Street, New York, NY 10017).

Figure 5.4. *Hospitals often use more than one light source for a given
spot as backup security in case one fails.*

strategy called Crime Prevention Through Environmental Design (CPTED), which was conceptualized more than 20 years ago by Oscar Newman in his book, *Defensible Space*. Since then, it has been validated by numerous studies and demonstrations sponsored by the National Crime Prevention Institute and the National Institute of Law Enforcement and Criminal Justice.

The basic idea behind CPTED is that the physical environment can be manipulated to produce effects that will reduce not only the incidence of crime but the *fear* of crime. These outcomes are accomplished by reducing the propensity of the physical environment to encourage criminal and negative behaviors. The three overlapping and interrelated components of CPTED are as follows:

Access control: Developing natural strategies for access control through spatial definition and traffic patterns. The purpose is to deny access to and challenge unwanted persons. Physical security includes locks, fences, gates, card access systems, and security personnel.

Surveillance strategies: Reducing or eliminating places for concealment. The purpose is to create an open environment where participants can see each other. Physical security includes bright lighting, low landscaping, windows, CCTV, clean building lines, and raised entryways/exits.

Territorial strategies: Making intruders feel unsafe and unwelcome with clear boundaries that make it obvious when they are trespassing. Clear property lines using fences, walls, and landscaping set up territory rights in the mind of the would-be intruder and serve as a deterrent.

These simple security planning and design considerations can prevent losses of significant value. Architects, designers, and security personnel should work together to create a safe and secure environment early in the security plan design process. It is far more cost effective to make architectural changes than to retrofit hardware or to have to use security personnel to manage security design flaws.

Applications for CPTED in the health care environment include the following:

Outpatient services. These should be located as close to building entry points as possible. It is also important to furnish telephones and toilet facilities in waiting areas to prevent persons from having to access other parts of the facility.

Fire exit emergency doors. These exit points should discharge internally to the campus, as opposed to the street, to make it difficult to load stolen property directly into a vehicle or to flee from a crime.

Trash processing area. Much more than garbage can easily go out with the trash, so dumpsters and compactors should be housed internally or located in a fenced and gated area. The person who processes the trash should not be able to hand materials to an accomplice or be able to access a vehicle easily from the processing area.

Parking structures. Avoid construction of internal stairwells and elevators; instead, use ones that are glassed in on three sides to provide for natural surveillance. Create vehicle entry and exit points internal to the campus. This configuration will not only keep street traffic from cutting through the garage as a shortcut, it will also reduce vehicle break-ins, vandalism, and even assaults.

Human resources. Do not place the human resources function in the main facility unless there is also an outside entrance to the employment office. This will reduce the number of job seekers wandering through the facility.

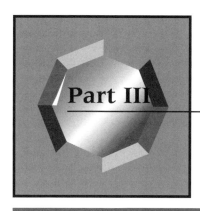

Part III

Security-Sensitive Areas

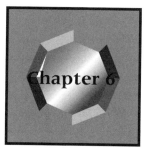

Chapter 6

Security
in the ED and ICU

D octor down, nurse and patient injured!" It sounds like a line from a made-for-TV movie. In fact, it is from a real-life scene being played out with increasing frequency in health care organizations in every part of the country. From simple assaults to homicides, workplace violence is a growing concern in physicians' offices, clinics, patient rooms, and trauma treatment areas, but nowhere more so than in the emergency department (ED). Often, all the prime ingredients of workplace violence come together in this one setting, the scene of approximately 50% of recorded incidents of aggressive action on medical center campuses.

The potential for violence travels a direct route between the ED and the intensive care unit (ICU) of a hospital. The victim of a gunshot wound, for example, typically is in the ED for a few minutes, goes right into surgery, and then lands in the ICU for an extended period of time—more than enough time for a renewal of hostilities by the perpetrator or his allies. Such a reprise of the original confrontation is a continuing risk for the patient and for his or her caregivers.

A study at the University of California, Irvine, Medical Center found that 686 episodes of emergency department violence occurred in one year.[3] When adjusted for the number of patients

treated, the study indicated that the greater percentage of these
violent incidents occurred on the night shift. (See Figure 6.1.)
The same study showed that the main treatment area of the ED
accounted for 336 reported incidents, or 49% of the total. Three
years later, a survey of 5,000 ED managers by the Emergency
Nurses Association revealed that 87% were exposed to physical
violence between one and five times a year; 24% had been
assaulted with weapons and 18% lost work time because of their
injuries.[4]

■ *Major Causes of ED Violence*

There are seven major conditions or causes of ED violence.
Usually, more than one is involved in a given incident.

Drug and alcohol influence. The drug impaired are frequent participants in ED violence. This includes visitors as well as

**LOCATION OF VIOLENT INCIDENTS WITHIN THE EMERGENCY
DEPARTMENT**

Main treatment area	49.0%
Custody/psychiatry room	29.2%
Triage/waiting room	17.8%
Ambulance ramp	4.0%
Total	100%

Source: Pane G, Salness K, Winiarski A, 1991, Aggression directed toward emergency department
staff at a university teaching hospital, *Annals of Emergency Medicine* 20(3): 283–86 Mar.

Figure 6.1.   *Together these four areas account for half of all violent
incidents in today's hospitals.*

patients and sometimes, although infrequently, staff. Alcohol leads the list of drugs involved in these episodes.

Gun proliferation. The number of guns in public possession is at an all-time high—an estimated 201 million in 1990, and that number rises yearly. More and more of these are automatic and semiautomatic weapons, which inflict greater physical damage and cause a parallel increase in the cost of medical care. A 1992 study of trauma patients treated in an Oakland, California, medical care facility found that the 15% of patients who were treated for gunshot wounds accounted for 44% of blood transfused. In another study, conducted at San Francisco General Hospital from 1991 to 1993, 80% of gunshot victims returned within three years with a similar wound; half of them were back within a year.[5]

Guns in hospitals are a major security concern. The American Medical Association has called on hospitals, the Joint Commission, and the American Hospital Association to adopt specific policies regarding this issue.

Decreased resources for mental health care. Funding for mental health care has been severely slashed over the past several years. Persons who were previously receiving care in a variety of inpatient and outpatient treatment programs are going without, or they are receiving substantially reduced treatment interventions. Many of these persons are showing up in emergency departments, at serious risk of injuring themselves or others.

Gang activity. Communities that thought themselves immune from gangs are being abruptly disabused of this notion. Gangs and gang activity are responsible for a significant amount of violence on the health care campus, not as a rule directed toward the organization but erupting in relation to the medical treatment of gang members.

Facility overcrowding. Treating 30,000 patients a year in an emergency department designed to treat 20,000 invites security incidents. As in clinics and ICU settings, overcrowding tends to be most acute in the waiting area, which is often squeezed into increasingly less space to accommodate increased patient treatment volume.

Unrealistic patient and staff expectations. Often, ED staff and patients have very different expectations of treatment outcomes and what it will take to achieve them. Patients (and their families and friends) expect instant and individualized care, regardless of the severity of their need. Staff expect patients to be extremely compliant and understanding of the complexities involved in the ED operation. The resulting clash can lead quickly to anger, the number one cause of security incidents between and among staff, patients, and visitors.

Lack of communication. No one likes to think he or she is being ignored. Yet that is exactly what thousands of emergency department patients and visitors think every day. Focused on medical treatment, busy staff all too often fail to properly communicate with patients and visitors—and when they do, their manner may cause further anger, leading to a violent incident.

The patient is the most common perpetrator of violence in the ED, the visitor in the ICU. When patients react negatively to a stressful event, it is most often in an attempt to gain control over their fear, anxiety, and feelings of being threatened. The same may be true of visitors, but sometimes a visitor is acting in a planned manner to retaliate against a staff member or patient for events—such as domestic disputes and gang activity—unrelated to medical issues; their actions may involve taking a hostage, kidnapping, or robbery.

Just as the patient can become angry during the treatment process, so too can staff members, who may at times exhibit behavior that contributes to the escalation of tension.

■ *Proactive Steps to Reducing Violence*

An act of violence can be committed by anyone at almost any-time. Yet sudden, unpredictable assault is really quite rare, compared to the number of assaults preceded by warning signs of one kind or another, such as these shown in Figure 6.2. It is generally accepted that the best predictor of violent behavior is past aggression, which is why some hospitals now flag the computer records of patients with a history of violence to alert ED and other staff. (See Figure 6.3.)

This discussion on reducing violence in the ED has focused on the patient. However, the same basic techniques apply to the visitor. The idea is to stay at least one step ahead of a violent act by quickly applying countermeasures at the first sign of danger;

WARNING SIGNS OF INCREASING ANGER/VIOLENCE

Pacing/restlessness

Clenched fist

Increasingly loud speech

Excessive insistence

Cursing

Quick movements/easily startled

Threats

Figure 6.2.   *Experienced ED personnel take these signs as cues to intervene sooner rather than later.*

GENERAL PROFILE OF VIOLENCE-PRONE PERSONS

Primarily male

Teens to mid-thirties

Unmarried

Low academic achievement

Lower socioeconomic class

Mental illness/chemical dependency

History of violence

Gang membership

Figure 6.3. *A history of violence is the most significant element in this profile.*

these measures include verbal, social, physical, and pharmaco-logic interventions.

Verbal and social interventions are closely interrelated and call for the caregiver and, when appropriate, friends and family, to assume an advocacy role on behalf of the disturbed patient. It is important to maintain an arms-length distance during dialogue and to indicate by positioning that he or she is in no way confined. Offering food, drink, and reassuring information often is all that is needed to reduce anxieties to acceptable levels. If de-escalation of the evident behavior does not occur, then it is time to set some limits in a firm but dispassionate manner: Tell the person what appropriate behavior is expected and that, for example, threatening actions will not be tolerated. At this point, additional staff should be alerted; the presence of a second caregiver may be helpful.

Setting limits leads naturally into a technique of maintaining control through "social contracting," which simply means that each party agrees to a specific outcome in exchange for certain actions and behaviors. Such a contract between a patient and caregiver might specify that a visitor would be allowed in the treatment room in exchange for patient cooperation. A visitor who is demanding to go into a treatment area to find out what is going on with a patient may be satisfied to sit down in the waiting area if the staff member promises to check on the patient and report back concerning his or her status.

When verbal intervention does not appear to be working, the next step is to prepare to restrain the patient physically. These are drastic steps, that should be taken with clinical justification and clear criteria to understand if they should be taken at all.

■ *The Security Officer and the ED*

In response to escalating violence, security officers are being seen more often in and around the emergency department. Note that this is not in itself the solution to the problem. In fact, the presence and actions of security may dilute or even discourage some of the other, equally important proactive measures, such as good staff practices and use of physical security, needed to maintain a safe and secure environment. The intervention of security personnel, especially if untrained, too early in the de-escalation process can precipitate rather than prevent violence. The caregiver who, instead of applying good coping skills to potentially troublesome situations, calls for security intervention at the drop of a hat is placing the entire staff and the organization at risk.

Although the use of off-duty police in a security role does not always yield the intended results, the extremely busy ED is one place where it may be necessary or advisable to use an off-duty police officer to supplement the in-house security effort. In these cases, the officer should be thoroughly educated on his or her role; any misunderstanding about the assignment can stir up rather than calm troubled waters. For example, while a patient who is acting out may technically be breaking a law, an arrest may not be in the best interests of medical care or the health care organization, which may well have a tolerance for disruptive behavior different than and beyond that of the police officer, whose authority supersedes hospital protocol.

There is significant misuse of security personnel in general in the typical emergency department, more so with the significant downsizing by hospitals: The better trained the security officers, the more helpful and resourceful they prove themselves to be, and the greater the number of inappropriate requests for their assistance. Especially in the ED, assistance with patients may even be contraindicated.

Security intervention in the ED is often called the "patient watch." The security officer is asked to maintain watch over a patient to avoid "tying up" a department caregiver or to avoid the application of physical restraints. There are various management problems associated with the security patient watch, not the least of which is the amount of time consumed. A patient watch often lasts for hours and may even extend over multiple shifts. In the meantime, the officer is not available to retrieve patient valuables from safekeeping, relieve a parking lot cashier, unlock a storeroom area, help a visitor with lost keys, escort an employee making a cash deposit, or carry out any number of other, proactive security duties and services. It is mandatory that a detailed protocol be developed concerning security policy and procedures relative to the patient watch, starting with a statement that makes it absolutely clear who has the authority to order and release security personnel from this type of assistance.

The appropriate use of security personnel to help maintain a safe environment in the emergency department may take the form of a random patrol of the area with response to called-for service or the posting of an officer in the ED either around the clock or for certain periods of the day. In general, security officers patrolling the ED are concerned with entrances, exits, waiting areas, ambulance driveway, triage, and, infrequently, the treatment areas. Timely support to these security-sensitive areas includes general surveillance of patients and visitors to spot impending trouble, standing by in a potentially violent situation, maintaining access control, and directly intervening in threatening situations.

Security interventions fall into two categories: intervention with patients, which is a collaborative effort with caregivers, and intervention with visitors and staff, which is undertaken independently. As a rule, the security officer should intervene with a patient only at the explicit or tacit request of a caregiver and under his or her direction. Of course, there are times when a caregiver is not present and a situation develops that requires immediate and independent action: when a patient who has not yet been treated, for example, suddenly "goes wild" in a waiting area, destroying property or posing a clear danger to himself or others, or when a security officer observes a patient dressed only in a gown attempting to leave through a fire exit door. In the case of a visitor or staff member who is acting out to the degree that security must intervene, the officer takes full charge and may request help and intervention from a caregiver in the immediate area.

Officers should always remain detached from the treatment being given to a patient. In one instance, a security officer reported that "while patrolling the corridor, he heard sounds of distress coming from the treatment room and entered to see if he could be of help." Upon entering, he noted a female patient twisting, turning, and uttering sounds of pain. He stated that he was holding her so she would not fall off the gurney while he was calling for assistance. The patient later alleged that the security officer fondled her.

Security officers should also refrain from rendering an opinion of the medical care. Telling a patient or family that they should not have to wait so long or that a treatment is not appropriate is strictly prohibited. If a security officer feels that an action truly is inappropriate, he or she should report it through the regular reporting structure of the organization.

◼ *Planning and Procedures*

Successful intervention either to prevent or physically stop disruptive or violent behavior is something that must be planned for. It is clearly the caregiver's responsibility to assume the leadership role in planning for the disruptive patient. Medical and administrative personnel share equally the responsibility for planning, policy, and procedures having to do with disruptive visitors, while administration, often the human resources department, is primarily responsible for planning relative to the disruptive employee.

In all interactions concerning potential or actual disruptive behavior, there will be a primary intervenor—on a nursing unit, for example, this is likely to be a nurse—with backup or support intervention provided in most cases by security, in extreme cases by police. But if the presence of security does not help, or if the behavior escalates, security then would assume primary responsibility for the situation. And if police do need to be called, security, in turn, would pass the responsibility on to them.

Most organizations also provide for a team response to severe situations, a strategy that may be very effective in a small facility that does not have a security response capability. The makeup of this team depends on the availability of personnel on each shift; it may or may not include caregivers. In facilities with large numbers of mental health and emergency medical technicians, team membership may be drawn entirely from this group. In other cases, maintenance, engineering, or environmental services personnel may serve. Response time is a major consideration in the development of this team, which typically is summoned by overhead or selective (beeper) paging.

There is no room to rely on instincts and let leadership simply emerge in dealing appropriately with disruptive behaviors in the health care organization. The role and expectations of participants must be carefully defined and thoroughly communicated upfront; to do otherwise is to risk finger pointing and other undesirable outcomes. It is generally agreed that interventions should use only the degree of force necessary to control the situation. Yet in case after case, critics—often led by the caregiver whose primary intervention was not successful—charge that either not enough force or too much force was applied. In one case, statements were taken from four caregivers concerning the actions of a security officer who, it was alleged, used too much force to handle a combative patient. One witness indicated that not enough force was applied and that it was applied too slowly, two felt the actions were appropriate, and one thought there had been excessive force.

Once policies and procedures establishing authority, responsibility, and role expectations have been written, the next step is to train those involved in their use. Some of this training will be in individualized groups of nurses, security personnel, or mental health workers. At some point, however, it will be necessary to bring all the participants together for group training exercises, which should include role playing. Training should be ongoing and include a review of each incident that takes place. In the wake of a major incident, a critical incident review team should perform an "audit" type of review, closely examining the action step by step, with an eye toward any modification in procedures or training that may be necessary, even if the outcome was positive.

■ *Physical Security Controls*

Physical security controls, including layout and design, are critical elements in protecting the emergency department. The basic objective of these controls is to maintain proper access control, establish protective barriers, and provide a simple and rapid means of summoning help; the degree to which they are applied will depend on the risk involved. The risk of violence is certainly greater in a level one trauma center that is located in a high crime area and treats 75,000 patients a year than in small facilities in safer areas.

Small or large, the layout and design of the ED should allow for the separation of at least four distinct containment areas: waiting and admissions, triage, treatment, and a holding room. For example, patients and visitors should not be able to access the treatment area freely from the waiting area or through a back entrance.

Figure 6.4 shows the layout of a simply designed emergency department in which there are six doors either always locked or capable of being locked.

Door 1 is the main ambulatory entrance, which is open 24 hours a day but equipped with a locking mechanism in case a total lockdown of the department is required.

Door 2 is the ambulance entrance, which should be locked 24 hours a day with controls at the nursing station.

Door 3 is the rear door to the department, which connects with the main part of the hospital. Patients going to surgery or to access other facility services would use this door, as would staff coming and going to other areas of the hospital. It

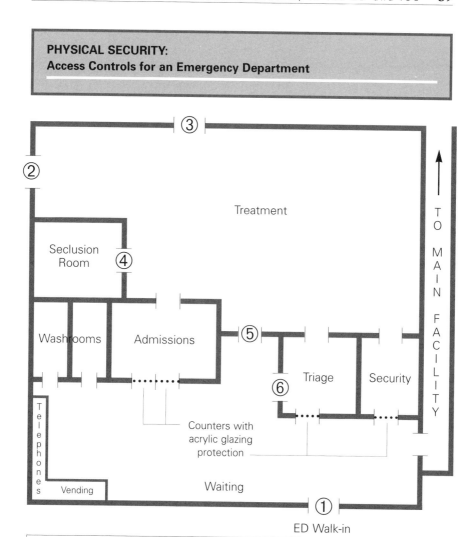

PHYSICAL SECURITY:
Access Controls for an Emergency Department

Treatment

TO MAIN FACILITY

Seclusion Room ④

Washrooms   Admissions   ⑤

Triage   Security

⑥

Telephones

Counters with acrylic glazing protection

Vending

Waiting

① ED Walk-in

Key: Numbers indicate doors equipped with locks

Figure 6.4. *As shown here, treatment, waiting, and triage areas should be separated from one another by locked doors.*

should be locked to restrict entry into the treatment area 24 hours a day.

Door 4 is the door to the holding room, which is locked only when occupied by a patient needing to be secluded.

Door 5 is a locked door that separates the treatment area from the waiting and admissions area.

Door 6 is a locked door to the triage area.

Note that the triage nurse and admissions personnel access their areas from the treatment area to avoid exposure to visitors or patients in the waiting area.

In the typical scenario, patients present themselves at the triage window and the triage nurse admits them through door 6 from the waiting area. The triage nurse may then direct patients back out to the waiting area and admissions or take them directly to the treatment area. Patients waiting for treatment are called to the area by a nurse from door #5.

To secure these different areas, the typical emergency department uses a vast array of physical controls in a variety of combinations; these include locks, duress alarms, glazing, communication-devices, secure containers, signage, lighting, closed circuit television, and metal detectors. (See Chapter 5, for a more detailed discussion of these items.) Each control should have its own written objective and usage plan. For example:

Metal detectors/magnetometers. Walk-through metal detectors in health care facilities are used relatively infrequently but, when used correctly, afford a high level of protection against the entry of metal weapons into the department. The equipment is not considered expensive, although operation of this access control device is quite labor intensive. In the busy ED, it may require two security officers to efficiently and effectively screen persons entering. Departments that do not use a walk-through metal detector often have a hand held unit available for special circumstances.

Duress (panic) alarms. These alarms are typically installed in treatment rooms and other areas where staff may be working alone and require immediate assistance. This type of alarm is used to summon medical help and security. Most often, there will also be a panic button installed at the admissions desk for security purposes. Although most panic-alarm systems are simply push buttons, various devices can be worn or carried by staff. These require an extensive electronic tracking system to pinpoint the point of activation.

Closed-circuit television (CCTV). Television is frequently used in the ED for security purposes and sometimes for patient surveillance. A properly protected camera located in the seclusion room, in the main waiting area, or at the ambulance entrance is a good use of CCTV. These systems are typically monitored at the ED nursing station and/or the ED security post in large operations. Any use of CCTV in treatment areas must protect the patients' rights of privacy and confidentiality.

Secure containers. As a safety practice, there should be an appropriate number of secure containers located in the ED to store the weapons of responding police or security officers; they are also useful for storing weapons or other contraband removed from patients or visitors. The typical container will have a key in the lock that can only be removed when the container is locked and should be carried by the person using the container.

How much security is appropriate? "Not enough" is the implication whenever a serious security incident occurs. On the other hand, instituting an armed camp that interferes with efficient medical treatment and frightens off customers is not the answer. A fine line must be walked between security measures that help make people feel secure and measures that simply make people think they are in a dangerous environment. As with the entire medical campus, constant monitoring and evaluation of the risks in the ED and ICU are necessary to ensure the proper level of security.

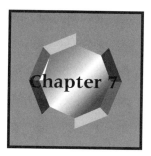

Chapter 7

Security
in Maternity
and Infant
Care Units

For an instant, the overhead page "Code Pink" brings normal hospital chatter and activity to a standstill. Within seconds, the staff is moving swiftly in reaction to a possible
infant kidnapping, with certain individuals performing specific
tasks, and others on the alert for anyone carrying a knapsack,
gym bag, or anything else that could conceal a baby.

Until the late 1980s, not much was known about the people
and methods involved in carrying out this worst nightmare of
new parents. There was no central collection of information
about the problem until the National Center for Missing and
Exploited Children (NCMEC) began asking questions about
infant abduction in 1983. The database created by the NCMEC
ultimately led to a national awareness of the problem and, more
importantly, to the creation of preventive guidelines for hospitals.
Together, these developments have been in large part responsible
for a dramatic reduction in this type of crime, from 12 to 15
abductions a year in the mid 1980s to 3 to 4 a year currently.
Between 1983 and 1995, a total of 88 infants were abducted in
36 different states; 5 are still missing.

The focus of the NCMEC in hospital-related work is the kidnapping of an infant (from birth to six months old) by a non-
family member. Kidnapping by a family member, while a much

more frequent occurrence and one that hospitals must guard against, is easier to resolve and generally has fewer negative consequences. In 1993, the U.S. Congress passed the International Parental Kidnapping Act to provide support in dealing with the domestic abduction problem, the full extent of which has yet to be documented.

■ *The Who and How of Infant Abductions*

The typical abductor appears to most to be a normal woman, often having given birth to at least one child and displaying all the characteristics of a loving mother. (See Figure 7.1.) She abducts a child not for ransom or for sale but, most often, to substitute for a baby she has lost or is unable to produce herself. The abducted infant is perceived by the abductor to be her own child, whose imminent arrival she has, in many cases, announced to family and coworkers. She may even have prepared a home nursery. Other abductors may act on impulse when faced with

---

TYPICAL PROFILE OF AN INFANT ABDUCTOR

Female of child-bearing age

Frequently impersonates a nurse or other caregiver

Demonstrates the capacity to provide good child care

Frequently tells others that she has lost a baby or is unable to have one

Usually lives in community where the abduction takes place

Generally is emotionally immature and has low self-esteem

Figure 7.1. *Women who steal infants often seem sincere rather than sinister.*

an unexpected opportunity or in an attempt to save a failing relationship. Some abductors work in tandem with a male cohort.

Typically, an abductor will have visited the birthing units of area hospitals, perhaps spending weeks or even months becoming familiar with the routine and layout of a facility, pretending to be a staff member, volunteer, or relative in friendly interactions with the mother of her intended target. Violence is not a part of the pattern; it is not necessary. Although 57% of babies are conned from their mothers in a postpartum unit, others are just as easily taken from staff in a nursery. The percentage of babies taken from specific locations within birthing units has remained consistent over the years. (See Figure 7.2.) Infants in pediatric units typically are taken from their beds when their parents are absent.

HOSPITAL INFANT-ABDUCTION LOCATIONS

Taken from	Number (Percent)
Mother's room	50 (57%)
Pediatrics	13 (15%)
Nursery	15 (17%)
Other areas of premises	10 (11%)
Total	100%

Source: National Center for Missing and Exploited Children, general memo, December 20, 1995.

Figure 7.2. *Obviously, vigilance must be the watchword wherever there are infants in hospitals.*

There have been no reported infant abductions from a hospital neonatal intensive care unit (NICU), although infants in the custody of a governmental family care agency or on "court hold" have sometimes been taken from the NICU by parents or relatives. The NICU environment presents certain security risks to which hospital staff must be particularly sensitive. Because infants often stay in the NICU for extended periods, they may have many more visitors than infants in normal birthing units. Also the intensive care nurse-to-patient ratio means many staff members are involved in an infant's care. The result is a lot of unfamiliar faces in a place from which hospital policy may permit direct discharge. During NICU hospitalization, an infant may receive numerous identification-band changes because of frequent IVs, edema, or a replacement for one that has slipped off. It is essential that the hospital have a clear policy and procedure on rebanding and matching identification at discharge. It is not always possible to reband the mother, who may have been discharged and is unavailable for a variety of reasons. In these cases the infant is often rebanded with a standard hospital identification band. (This type of situation can also occur in the well baby newborn nursery, and the same policy and procedures for rebanding and matching identification would be applicable.)

Knapsacks, backpacks, and gym bags are often used to conceal the victim of an abduction, although some babies have simply been carried in open view down a stairway and out the nearest door. Most abductors carefully plan their escape route but others have been known to get lost while trying to get out. In one case, an abductor made a wrong turn and ended up in an oncology unit; she appeared so out of place there that a visitor became suspicious and alerted staff, who arranged for her apprehension and the safe return of the baby.

The majority of infants are abducted during the day, when units are busiest and people can move about with more anonymity. There are sufficient exceptions to this generality, however, that a hospital cannot afford to relax security precautions at any hour of the day or night.

Infant Security Requirements

Facing the infant abductor are a number of security precautions developed by the NCMEC in concert with various governmental agencies, health care associations, and individual health care security experts. These measures can be separated into three categories: identification, education and training, and physical security safeguards.

Identification involves the infant, the mother, her significant other, and hospital caregivers who are allowed to transport the baby. Since the infant should be in the custody and control of either the mother or a staff member at all times, making sure each party knows to whom they are releasing the baby is a big part of the battle. For this reason, distinctive uniforms are insufficient to identify staff authorized to transport infants; these individuals must also wear what is called "secondary identification" in the form of a special badge or a regular staff ID badge modified in some special way.

The identification of the baby begins at the time of birth: Medical personnel do a physical assessment, obtain a blood specimen, and apply numbered ID bands identical to those worn by the mother. The four-band ID system, which is the most commonly used, provides two bands for the baby, one for the mother, and one for the person the mother designates as her significant other. Although the baby is still in the birthing room, or within two hours of birth, he or she should be footprinted and color photographed.

Even before the birth, however, the mother should be educated about security and safety practices in prenatal childbirth classes, preadmission facility tours, upon admission, and during postpartum instruction. At each point, the importance of identifying all persons handling and transporting her baby should be stressed. It is recommended that these instructions be in the form of a checklist, which the mother signs and which becomes part of the medical record. (See Figure 7.3.)

Staff security training is yet another element in the prevention of infant abductions. Staff must not only be knowledgeable in terms of security policy but be motivated to practice security procedures. They must be aware of the abductor profile, unusual

---

SAMPLE SECURITY INSTRUCTION CHECKLIST FOR MATERNITY PATIENTS

Keep your infant in your direct line of sight even when you go to the bathroom.

Close room door or preferably have nurse take your baby back to the nursery if you plan to sleep.

Become familiar with hospital staff and know the nurse(s) assigned to you and your baby.

Question unfamiliar persons entering your room even if they are wearing hospital attire; alert the nurses' station if you have any doubt about their presence.

Do not give your baby to anyone who does not have proper staff identification that has been explained to you.

Do not give out any information about you or your baby over the telephone or to anyone in person unless you absolutely know him or her.

Ask about any follow-up care to be provided by the hospital in your home and procedures for verifying the identity of the caregiver.

Figure 7.3. *A written checklist makes a stronger impression than any amount of verbal instruction.*

STAFF SECURITY AWARENESS REGARDING INFANT ABDUCTIONS

All staff members should be on the alert for

    Repeat visitors with extreme interest in "babies"

    Theft of uniforms or staff identification

    Extensive questions regarding infant-unit protocols

    Persons carrying infants instead of using a bassinet

    Persons carrying bags, large packages, or loosely wrapped bundles from the unit

Figure 7.4. *Any of these events should trigger suspicions.*

and suspicious behaviors, and the critical incident response plan. (See Figure 7.4.)

Physical Security Safeguards

The application of physical safeguards should be designed in consultation with a qualified professional on the basis of the specific layout of the facility and its general environmental and security vulnerabilities, as well as on nationally accepted guidelines concerning access control to vulnerable areas of the hospital and applicable state statutes.

Locking mechanisms are required in two specific areas of a maternity unit. First, all doors to all nurseries should be equipped with self-closing hardware and locked at all times; frequent entry by staff makes the nursery an excellent application for an electronic card access system. Second, there should be locking mechanisms on exit doors that lead directly outside and on exit doors to stairwells that lead outside. Locks are optional at the main entrances to postpartum and pediatric units and single-room maternity care areas.

In addition to being locked, exit doors require alarms and a closed-circuit television (CCTV) system to capture, on videotape, all persons leaving the unit. Alarms should sound at the door as well as at the nursing station and/or a central security monitoring station; use of a shunt will make it possible for staff to enter and exit through locked doors without activating the alarm. Consideration should also be given to monitoring the CCTV system at the nursing station and/or at the security office. Other applications of CCTV include the public entrance to the maternity unit, and any areas not in the direct line of sight of the nursing station, such as an elevator lobby. CCTV may also be used in programs with electric lock releases.

Electronic surveillance is increasingly used on maternity units. In such systems (often referred to as tag systems), a tag or similar device—attached to the infant's wrist, ankle, diaper, or umbilical cord—alerts staff via an alarm when its wearer is passing through a detection field. There are a number of different system designs, some of which are quite simple and some of which require staff to replace batteries, input computer data, and perform other administrative tasks.

All physical security systems should be identified and fully described in the security management plan, including use, goals, and objectives; they should be fully operational at all times. The inactive security system can be a detriment to the overall protection level of the organization; if a system is shut off, not in use, or broken and not being repaired immediately, it should be dismantled and removed. Whenever security is down (except during maintenance), staff must evaluate the need for temporary, supplemental and/or alternative safeguards, especially in security-sensitive areas.

■ *The Critical Incident Response Plan*

All facilities at risk for the abduction of infants or children must develop a written response plan specific to the type of patient involved. For example, the abduction of a pediatric or NICU patient may require locating the parent(s), who may not be present in the facility.

The plan should include a code word that is communicated to the entire hospital, generally by overhead page and radio, to alert staff to the possibility that an infant abduction has taken place. Many hospitals use "Code Pink." Nursing and security will be responsible for the primary initial response action.

Maternal/Child-Care Nursing Staff Guidelines during Infant-Abduction Alert

- Immediately notify security and/or other designated hospital authority. Begin complete unit search and do a head count of all infants.

- Protect the immediate area where the abduction occurred to preserve any forensic evidence.

- Brief other staff members on the situation and have them advise all mothers in the area (but only when mother and infant are together). It is important for mothers to be informed by staff of the problem rather than hearing it through other patients, the media, or law enforcement. Move the parents to a private room off the maternity floor and assign a nurse to stay with them at all times to provide support and protect them from stressful media contacts or other undue interferences.

- As soon as practical, proceed with group discussion sessions with affected hospital staff to assess and deal with post-traumatic stress disorder.

Security Staff Guidelines during Infant-Abduction Alert

- Immediately notify the police and as soon as possible the FBI and the NCMEC.

- Immediately begin an exterior search, securing the most common exit points and, to the extent possible, the remainder of the perimeter.

- Go to the abduction site to obtain pertinent information and to take responsibility for protecting the crime scene pending the arrival of law enforcement personnel.

- Maintain law enforcement liaison, brief facility spokesperson(s), help with the notification of media, and oversee control of reporters' activities on the property.

- Notify other appropriate health care facilities in the geographical area about the incident, providing a full description of baby and abductor.

Other organization resources that will play an important response role include public relations, switchboard personnel, and risk management.

Once written and taught to staff, the infant-abduction response plan should be evaluated and modified as necessary through periodic review and drills to ensure that the intended outcomes are, in fact, what results. The same general guidelines and principles should be applied to abductions from elsewhere on the hospital premises, including the pediatric unit.

Given the fact that maternity stays are becoming shorter, it is safe to assume that, in the future, home aftercare for new mothers will become an established part of a hospital's continuum of care; as such, it will require increased security attention by health care providers.

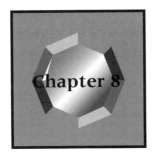

Security
in the Pharmacy

Drugs. All by itself, the word conjures visions of lawless behavior. The number of robberies and burglaries of hospital pharmacies is down, one reflection of how easy it is to obtain illicit drugs on the street these days—why take the relatively high risk of getting caught stealing from a pharmacy when street supplies are so plentiful? Drug diversions, however, are up. In this category of crime, no drugs are actually missing, per se; they are simply diverted: A nurse administers less of a drug than is prescribed, pocketing the rest; a physician substitutes saline solution or a sugar pill for the real thing.

It is generally recognized that there is a high degree of substance abuse among health care professionals, not least because they have so many opportunities to obtain drugs. (See Figure 8.1.) Not all health care workers who steal drugs do so for their own personal use, however. A large number of these thefts are for resale or are intended for a friend or significant other.

The stakes are not particularly high. Many cases that do result in criminal charges are plea bargained down to where they have a very low level of impact on the individual—and on the problem. A great many more cases are now being handled through drug rehabilitation programs, redefining the problem as medical rather than criminal. Often overlooked in drug

---

COMMON DRUG DIVERSIONS/THEFTS BY STAFF

Substituting a non-narcotic, in liquid form, for the legitimate narcotic

Altering or falsifying sign-out sheets or patient medication records

Falsifying a physician's order

Theft and substitution of unit-dose syringes

Theft from anesthesia and surgery units

Theft of narcotic sign-out sheets and remaining narcotics

Bogardus, D, 1994, *Missing Drugs II*, Gilbert, AZ: Medical Management Systems (P.O. Box 1582, Gilbert, AZ 85299–1582).

Figure 8.1.   *Unfortunately, some health care staff members abuse their access to pharmaceuticals.*

diversions is the suffering of the patient, who is forced to do without the medication designed to effect a cure or to relieve pain. This is a problem that deserves a closer look in the design of effective drug control.

▪ *The Pharmacy Defined*

In terms of security, *pharmacy* has a broad meaning. It includes not only the main hospital pharmacy and satellite pharmacies—the focus of security standards from the Joint Commission's perspective—but also clinics, nursing units, and any other points where controlled substances are stored or used. All of these come under the purview of the director of pharmacy or chief pharmacist, whose responsibility extends to the administration of the drug to the patient.

As with other security-sensitive areas, the restriction of unauthorized personnel is a primary security objective. Strict access control to the pharmacy requires that all access points be locked around the clock. The typical hospital pharmacy has two or three primary access points, including the service counter area, the staff entrance, and the product receiving door. In some cases the staff entrance and the product receiving door are one and the same. The mere locking of an area does not preclude the entry of an unauthorized person, who may wait in the corridor until an employee exits or follow behind an employee as he or she is entering. The service counter, for example, must be designed so a person cannot simply crawl over it. Furthermore, the pharmacy must be physically constructed to deter or detect a burglary. In one hospital, no one had checked to ensure that the pharmacy wall extended through the false ceiling to the floor above; a canny thief was able to remove a ceiling tile in the main corridor and climb over the wall into the pharmacy.

The Security Plan

As a designated security-sensitive area, the pharmacy must have a complete, written security plan. One component of this overall plan concerns access control implementation policies and procedures, which should cover the following:

- Hours of operation;

- Accountability for keys, cards, and lock combinations;

- Physical security controls in place; and

- Employee responsibilities regarding access controls.

Of particular concern is after-hours access to the pharmacy that does not operate on a 24-hour basis. Some employees may have both authorization to enter the pharmacy at night and a legitimate reason for doing so—for instance, the night nursing supervisor—and others may have only authorization, such as the pharmacy worker who returns after hours for not-so-legitimate reasons. In the case of the nursing supervisor, there is concern for his or her safety as well as for accountability of action. Security often performs an access role in accompanying such persons, including emergency maintenance personnel, into the pharmacy areas.

A common access control measure is the dual lock system, in which two different individuals, each supplying one-half of the control mechanism, must cooperate to gain entry. This can involve two different key locks, a reader control requiring two cards, or a combination of an access card and a key for a conventional lock.

A second component of the pharmacy security plan consists of policies and procedures for the use of preventive security measures, including the following:

- Transporting of drugs;

- Release of drugs;

- Compliance with control procedures;

- What to do in case of a robbery;

- Destruction of controlled substances;

- Loss-reporting procedures;

- Signs of drug diversion;

- Persons responsible for changing locks or combinations under certain conditions.

Although many of these security procedures are mandated by law, design and implementation of security measures to ensure the area's safety and security are the organization's responsibility.

Locks. The primary physical control of the pharmacy encompasses not only good locking mechanisms but establishing an entry audit trail: a record of who gained access, at what time, and on what date. The audit trail is extremely important for clinics, satellite units, and off-premises facilities, and also can be very useful in monitoring off-hours activities in the 24-hour pharmacy.

There is no substitute for a computer access control system that grants access to authorized persons during authorized time periods and records attempted activation during nonauthorized time periods. For example, a pharmacy employee who works Monday through Friday during the day would not be able to use a combination code or biometrics device to gain entry at night or on the weekends.

Alarms. There is widespread use of both intrusion and panic alarm systems in drug formulation, dispensing, and storage areas. The need for intrusion alarms for an area that is closed and locked during portions of the day is apparent. But there also are times in the 24-hour pharmacy when staff are not actually present, when an intrusion alarm can help ensure that no one has gained entry and is waiting inside for staff to return.

In facilities that have a security response capability, panic or duress alarms are often installed at the pharmacy service counter, remote work areas, and the narcotics vault, where they provide not only an efficient means of summoning help but an element of reassurance to staff.

Closed-Circuit Television (CCTV). Depending on layout and design, there are good applications for CCTV as part of the pharmacy protection plan. The two primary areas for CCTV cameras would be the main service window and the staff/receiving entry point. At the service window, the camera acts to deter crime and

to keep watch for staff who are away from the window performing other tasks; a sensor installed with the camera, or a service
bell, can alert staff that someone at the counter needs service.
The second and more important camera would view the corridor
outside the staff or receiving door, enabling staff about to exit the
pharmacy to see if there is any suspicious activity in the corridor.

Figure 8.2 shows two cameras and two monitors in a relatively simple application of CCTV. The monitor in the work area
provides a picture of both cameras, while the monitor at the
staff/receiving entry point sees only the corridor. A third monitor,
not shown, could be added to the service counter area to view
the staff receiving/entry corridor, as well, thus allowing staff to
observe someone seeking entry before electrically releasing the
door. This function could be performed from either the service
counter or the work area, if such a capability was part of the
access control plan

Any CCTV equipment installation must allow for video
recording of all cameras, ideally with a time-lapse recorder that
permits taping over an extended period. A time and date genera-
tor is desirable but not always necessary, depending on the objectives of the CCTV system. The access control plan should include
a tape retention schedule, with 72 hours before reuse the recommended minimum.

The Service Window.   The service window is the point of many
pharmacy transactions, whether service is aimed at inpatients
only or at the general public. During the past few years, such
transactions have declined with improvements in accountability
and the individual packaging of many medications. In fact, most
drugs, including narcotics, are stocked at the unit by pharmacy
employees, often making use of special dispensing units that provide for much tighter control of drugs.

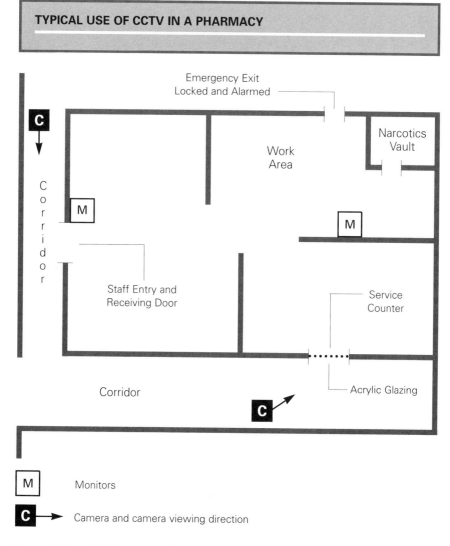

Figure 8.2. *CCTV cameras in the pharmacy should be recording at all times.*

The service window should be protected by acrylic glazing to protect staff from assault or robbery, with small openings to facilitate communication and dispense small items. A pass-through door or revolving, lazy Susan-type platform can be installed for larger items. If the pharmacy service window is not used during a portion of the day, a metal or heavy wood door should close off the window opening.

There should be no entry door to the pharmacy located immediately adjacent to the service window unless there is a wall partition between door and window to break the line of sight. This eliminates the scenario that played out in one small southern hospital, where a robber managed to extend his arm—and the gun at the end of it—through the service window opening, point the gun at the pharmacy technician, and order her to unlock the adjacent door; had he not been able to keep his weapon trained on her the whole time, she might have been able to summon help. Very small openings at the service counter also may preclude such use of a weapon. However, many counters use larger openings to accommodate routine transactions during the day.

■ *Pharmacy Staff*

The theft of controlled substances and other drugs from pharmacies continues to be a major security problem for health care organizations. This involves primarily pharmacy employees, from clerk to registered pharmacist, but there also are instances of delivery, maintenance, and environmental services staff taking advantage of an uncontrolled situation to help themselves to drugs.

It is essential to thoroughly check and evaluate the background of any applicant for employment in the hospital pharmacy. The thief who plans to learn the system meticulously while employed by the pharmacy is a fact of life as well as a staple of fiction. And such thieves are often successful. In Minnesota, a pharmacist pleaded guilty to federal charges of theft after allegedly taking thousands of dollars worth of prescription drugs from the hospital where she worked to sell at a retail pharmacy she and her husband owned. In Milwaukee, a pharmacy clerk responsible for ordering and stocking shelves was charged with diverting up to 150 tablets a day. Such crimes are not always solo acts. In Georgia, police investigating the theft of controlled substances arrested two people: the assistant director of the pharmacy and a staff pharmacist.

Once screened and checked for employment, pharmacy staff become a first line of defense against drug diversions. The Joint Commission specifically requires hospitals to educate and train staff in security-sensitive areas in basic security practices, both when they are first hired and as an ongoing management process. Staff should be alert at all times to the conduct of anyone involved in the administration of drugs.

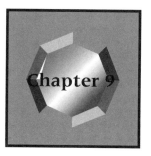

Chapter 9

Security in Parking Facilities

renda, a nurse at Memorial Hospital, was at the end of a 12-hour shift. It was 3 AM and she was tired. She didn't want to "waste time" calling for a security escort, which would delay her departure at least five minutes. If she should need assistance, she knew there were emergency call stations, marked by a blue light, on the way to the parking lot. And so Brenda decided to go it alone and did, indeed, arrive home five or seven minutes earlier than if she had requested an escort.

Were those few minutes worth the risk? The answer seems obvious—no. Had Brenda run into serious trouble on the way to her car, she no doubt would have said the same thing herself afterward—if she had been able to talk. And yet hospital employees will generally elect convenience over safety. Most of the time, everything turns out all right.

Campus parking areas are a major concern for security in terms of both personal safety and property loss or damage. Between 1995 and 1996, a physician was carjacked in New Mexico, a purse snatcher ended up killing a cancer patient in the parking garage of a Baltimore hospital, and a female medical student was assaulted returning to her car outside a hospital in Illinois. All three incidents occurred between 4:30 PM and 6:30 PM; further proof of what security officers already know very well: Not all serious parking lot security incidents occur during the dead of night.

Even though parking lots are a major concern and receive a good deal of security attention, they are only infrequently considered a security-sensitive area. In fact, the parking areas of a health care facility present a very high risk of premises liability.

The key factors in evaluating the security risk potential of the parking site is its location, its history of security problems, and its designated use during high-risk hours. For example, a specific parking area may present a low security risk during the day but an extremely high one at night. Because the demand for parking is considerably less at night, the security solution to this problem may be to simply shut the area and limit parking to specific daytime hours.

Because of the lack of land on which to expand surface lots, the multilevel parking structure has become a way of life on most health care campuses. Although either type of parking arrangement can be basically safe or unsafe, the vast majority of people *feel* safer in a surface lot—assuming of course, that it is not located in a very remote, dark, high-crime area. This is primarily because of the line of sight. The proper design of a structure can do a great deal to counter the closed-in feeling that many parking garages seem to generate.

■ *Securing the Surface Parking Area*

Prime considerations for securing the surface parking area are access control and landscaping. Access control in this context refers to minimizing foot traffic through the area, as well as controlling which vehicles are allowed access to specific areas. Much vehicle vandalism and break-ins can be avoided by diverting pedestrians who would otherwise use the lot as a short cut.

The most common deterrents to foot traffic are barriers (even partial barriers), the geographic placement of the parking area, and good signs. The use of berms, shrubs, and well-defined and convenient walkways is always helpful. Controlling access with a barrier does not always mean fencing the entire parking area using chain-link fencing with barbed wire outriggers. A barrier on one side of the parking area—for example, shrubbery, or shrubbery combined with fencing—may be all that is needed to redirect a traffic pattern. In high-risk surface areas, it may be necessary to "harden the target" with complete fencing, card access, and closed-circuit television (CCTV).

Proper landscape design and maintenance of a parking area can eliminate three security problems: a limited line of sight, hiding places for persons or property, and improperly trimmed foliage that cuts into the effectiveness of night lighting. For this reason, scheduled nighttime inspections of the landscape should be conducted at staggered intervals, to gauge the effect of plants and trees in all seasons. This type of inspection makes an excellent security performance standard.

Closed-Circuit Television.   The use of CCTV for general security surveillance in parking lots has limited cost-effectiveness. To mount cameras on poles, electrical power and coaxial cable connections are needed. Outdoor camera housings, which may require heating units are also needed. All this is less expensive when there are adjacent buildings where cameras can be mounted; using the pan, tilt, and low-light camera configuration, it is possible to scan a large area with a roof-mounted camera. But the cost of the equipment, installation, and, most important, live monitoring, is still very high.

Observation Posts.   The use of an attended observation post in a parking area is a common and effective element of the protection system and one that enhances the feeling of security among parking lot users. Such a post can be staffed either regularly during certain hours or randomly. It can also serve as a shelter against the elements for patrolling security officers. The post should be put where there is the widest and clearest view, but away from the perimeter of the lot if the safety of the officers is an issue. Its floor should be least two feet above the grade, or ground level, of the lot.

Emergency Call Stations.   Hospitals are beginning to follow the lead of colleges and universities in installing emergency call stations on the campus grounds, including parking areas. Typically identified by a blue light and appropriate signage, these stations are placed so they are visible from almost any location on the campus.

When the call station communication device is activated, a strobe light begins flashing and continues to do so for a specific period of time. The purpose of the strobe light is to frighten off a would-be assaulter or harasser while guiding responding security personnel. The communication devices connect directly with a switchboard operator or security dispatcher, and the signal automatically indicates which call station has been activated.

Although these stations are commonly referred to as emergency communication devices, they often serve a broader purpose. A system recently installed on the campus of a major hospital in Denver displays the word *HELP* in big letters as a beacon to people who have locked themselves out of their cars, have a flat tire, or simply need directions.

■ *Securing the Parking Structure*

The multilevel parking garage presents a different set of security considerations. Chief among these are a much more restricted line of sight and the addition of stairwells and elevators, each of which creates areas of concealment, as well as a more closed-in feeling.

A great deal can be done to decrease this feeling. A design that creates long lines of sight and provides for maximum amount of openness to the outside is a good place to begin, followed by cleanliness and light. In this sense, light means not only natural daylight and electrical lights but the interior surfaces of the structure; columns, ceilings, curbs, and walls should all be painted white or another light color to enhance the electrical lighting.

Stairwells and Elevators.   Stairwells and elevators of the parking structure are most vulnerable to assaults and purse snatches. A stairwell in particular offers concealment and a quick exit for the transgressor. An excellent countermeasure is to design glass-enclosed stairwells, which are highly visible to persons outside the building. The same is true for elevators: A glass-enclosed shaft on the exterior of the structure, with a glass-enclosed elevator cab, has become a common security design feature of parking structures.

Persons should be able to access the stairwell at ground level only from within the garage. The emergency exit to the street should be locked and alarmed.

Emergency Call Stations, Panic Alarms, and CCTV.   For summoning assistance, the parking structure should have the same voice-activated emergency call stations as the surface parking areas as well as conveniently placed panic buttons. The panic buttons should be located in conspicuous locations on each floor and in stairwells, with emphasis on the word *conspicuous*. Too often, these devices go completely unnoticed. A large background painted a contrasting color, large lettering, and lighting are all helpful additions to the emergency call station.

The primary application for CCTV in the parking lot is at vehicle access points and elevator/stairwell areas where emergency call stations are located. (See Figure 9.1.) In some systems, a CCTV camera will scan a large general area but "lock on" to the emergency call station area when the station is activated.

The cashier booth is a good location for security monitoring devices in facilities large enough to staff such booths around the clock. Back-up or alternative locations for these devices can be elsewhere on the campus or even across town in a dedicated monitoring facility.

Surveillance Potential.   All parking areas, including surface lots and multilevel structures, require covert surveillance occasionally, if not often, typically in the wake of a rash of vehicle break-ins, assaults, stolen vehicles, vandalism, or threats of various kinds. A van parked in the target area, with dark tinted glass and a security officer or investigator inside, serves very well in these instances. Permanent surveillance areas may even be created within a parking structure, such as in an enclosed storage area or machine room that allows for installation of one-way window glass. This design concept should be considered during the planning stages of the structure, but retrofitting can generally be accomplished with minimal expense.

■ *Common Parking Security Considerations*

Surface lots and parking garages each have unique security needs, as well as many common safeguards. The most important need in each is for adequate security patrols and a rapid security response capability. Patrol frequency and fixed post assignments are dictated by the degree of vulnerability each area has to the gamut of security risks. In all cases, a clean, well-maintained

TYPICAL SECURITY APPLICATIONS IN A PARKING STRUCTURE

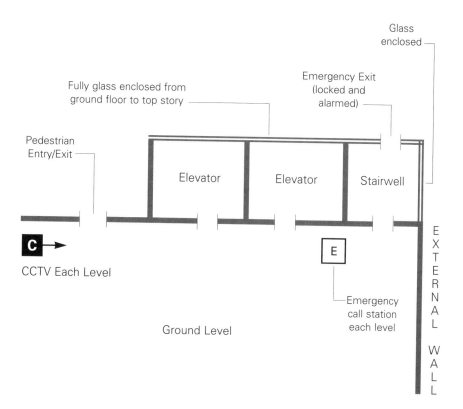

Figure 9.1. *Cameras trained on emergency call stations allow security personnel to zero in on problems the instant they occur.*

environment is important in promoting a safe feeling among users and in discouraging negative behaviors.

Security escort service is highly promoted on most health care campuses. But although the employee is generally quite aware of this service, extra effort is required to inform visitors and patients of its availability. Security is normally deployed in parking areas during major shift changes, when employees are encouraged to leave work in groups rather than requesting individual escorts.

It is arriving staff who are the more vulnerable, and the best security parking plan for afternoon and night shifts designates specific parking areas for these employees. Concentrating the parking of vehicles makes patrol and surveillance more effective and makes staff feel safer. Since signs by themselves are typically insufficient to control parking, particularly where there is a shortage of spaces, security will have to physically block off and open these designated areas at specific times.

The primary entry/exit of a parking area, for both pedestrians and vehicles, should be internal to the campus rather than lead directly to the street. (See Figure 9.2.) The secondary exit points shown would be gated to maintain the security integrity of the area and opened during periods of heavy outgoing traffic. The street side of the area may also be protected by fencing or the wall of the parking structure. Particular attention should be given to the grade level of a parking structure, so that a pedestrian cannot simply walk in or crawl over a low wall or fence.

Parking Shuttle Vehicles.   As a health care campus expands, there may be a need to establish remote or off-site parking areas for staff. Shuttle vehicles are commonly used to provide transportation to and from these areas. Having uniformed security personnel drive these vehicles has proven to be highly effective in terms both of protecting parked vehicles and of staff satisfaction, since these personnel can simultaneously provide a security patrol function. In some programs, shuttles are clearly marked as security/escort vehicles, providing yet another visible element of protection.

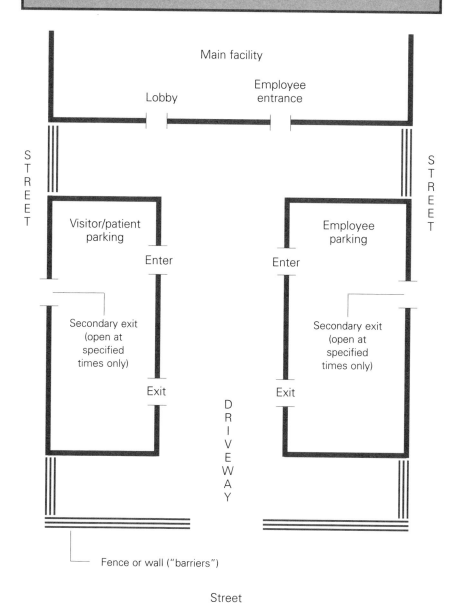

Figure 9.2. *Direct access to the street from parking lot or garage should be tightly controlled at all times.*

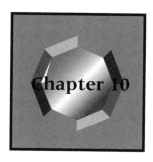

Chapter 10

Facility-Specific Security Risks

A rson by animal rights activists and assaults by psychiatric patients are not major concerns at every hospital, but in some places they receive high priority on the security agenda. In addition to the common security-sensitive areas already discussed, a hospital may have specific functions and activities that officials wish to designate security sensitive in acknowledgement of particularly high levels of risk. Medical records, medical research, and satellite clinics are all candidates for such status, depending on their situation within a facility.

Medical Records

Unauthorized release of medical record information clearly would put a health care organization and its staff at risk for civil and even criminal liability. Unfortunately, reports of confidential patient information being sold by hospital employees are not unusual, and outright theft of such information occurs with alarming frequency. Clearly, it is of great value to a variety of people, including those involved in litigation and, more benignly, marketers interested in a specific patient population.

Over the course of an average admission, 75 or more persons may have legitimate access to a patient's medical record; what they cannot remember they can easily copy, thanks to the prolif-eration of copy machines.

The legitimate release of medical records is contingent on three factors: the consent of the individual to whom the record pertains; a subpoena or court order; and the requirement to report certain information to agencies specified by law, such as information pertaining to infectious diseases and child abuse. The sheer volume of requests for medical records is staggering—up to more than 300,000 per year for one organization, according to testimony from large providers before the U.S. Senate's Privacy Protection Study Commission several years ago.[6]

Protection of the medical record rests with the caregiver until a patient is discharged, after which the security of the record—including storage, copying, access, and release of information—is the direct responsibility of the medical records department.

Access Control.   A major security concern relative to the medical records department is access control:

- Can nondepartment staff, gain free access to the working areas of the department during regular business hours? Can strangers?

- How are records accessed by staff after hours?

- Can physicians who come in to "clean up" their charts gain access to the dictation area at all times? Can the main working and storage areas be accessed from the dictation area?

- Are records secured in remote storage locations? How safe are staff in accessing these locations after hours?

- How sound is the physical security of the area in terms of locks and alarms?

Most medical records departments will need the resources of a security professional to adequately address these questions and to help formulate the security plan. Security support for this area should include staff education on proper security procedures, proper locking and alarming, and providing or monitoring after-hours access. A card access system integrated with intrusion alarms is highly recommended.

Personal Safety.   Personal safety during regular business hours is not generally regarded as a significant security problem in the medical records department, but the same cannot be said for small numbers of staff or persons working alone in fairly remote areas of the facility during off-hours. Such areas should be secured and supported by frequent security patrols, augmented by the use of fixed panic alarms or the kind that can be worn by employees. Security escorts or a policy requiring two persons to access remote storage locations during off-hours is recommended.

■ *Cashiers*

The cashier function presents a multitude of security risks, from armed and unarmed robberies to embezzlement, theft by deception (short-change artists, bad checks), threats, and assaults. An armed robbery is most likely to occur in parking areas, including surface lots and multilevel structures; however, the hospital's main cashier and the pharmacy cashier are both vulnerable targets.

Few cashier operations are impervious to a determined embezzler. There is generally always a way to beat the system, and individual cashiers will go to great lengths to figure it out. (See Figure 10.1.)

THE CASHIER VS THE SYSTEM

Embezzlers can too easily

    Not ring the sale and pocket the amount

    Underring the sale and pocket the difference

    Perform one's own reconciliation of funds

    Underring sales for friends

    Give phony refunds

    Make fraudulent overring corrections

Figure 10.1. *Victim or victimizer, the cashier represents a vulnerable spot in the system.*

The cashier who is working in a public area should be protected by a security-designed safety window; the door to his or her work station should be locked. Where this is not feasible, as in many gift shops and cafeterias, other physical security measures become more important, such as panic alarms and closed-circuit television systems. Additional control procedures include maintaining minimal amounts of cash, providing adequate escort service, and educating cashiers regarding crime prevention. Risk levels should be separately evaluated for each hour of business.

■ *Medical Research*

Medical research poses a major security risk, one that is heightened by the use of animals. Animal-rights activists are considered dangerous in the pursuit of their cause and rightly so: An analysis of incidents occurring in 1993 found that the most frequent criminal tactic used by these groups was nonpeaceful protests followed by arson and vandalism.[7] Compared to previously collected data, this study suggested that nonpeaceful protests are increasing significantly. And health care and pharmaceutical companies that conduct consumer product testing are second only to hunting clubs in terms of animal-rights incidents. An extreme example of such activity occurred in 1989 at the University of Arizona, where the Animal Liberation Front broke into three laboratory facilities and caused more than $100,000 in damage through fire and vandalism, in addition to releasing more than 1,000 research animals.

There is, of course, considerable medical research in health care facilities that does not involve animals. The greatest security risk to such operations is the disgruntled staff member or the employee who has been terminated for cause. The most serious forms of retaliation are altered or stolen research data and destruction of equipment and substances relating to research in progress, acts that are typically not preceded by threats. In fact, a person who makes open threats of this type is unlikely to carry them out. Still, each and every threat must be taken seriously.

The most important security measures for research areas are strict access control procedures, physical separation of research activity, and back-up storage of critical data (redundancy). The very nature of research requires that staff have 24-hour access to facilities, and it is not uncommon for researchers to work all night or return after hours to monitor or adjust an experiment. Obviously, it is important to know which persons will be accessing which areas at which times.

Behavioral Health Care

Despite security precautions, patients being treated for behavioral or substance abuse problems in the emergency department, the outpatient clinic, or the open or closed inpatient unit necessitate frequent interventions by security personnel. It is not uncommon for medical staff to be assaulted by a mentally impaired person during treatment, and more often, such patients are returning to treatment facilities after discharge expressly to cause disruption and even bodily harm.

In one case, a patient who had been seen with some regularity at a Missouri facility returned to the facility late at night. Parking his vehicle in the ambulance driveway, he took a weapon from the trunk, entered the emergency department through the ambulance entrance, and shot and killed a physician and a visitor. Elsewhere, a middle-aged woman calmly entered a Michigan hospital and began shooting, seriously wounding two technicians; she later explained that she thought they were doctors and that she blamed doctors for the death of her mother five years earlier.

One function of health care security officers is to help caregivers handle disturbed patients, whether they are psychiatric patients or general patients disoriented as a result of medication. Such assistance is generally in response to a call for service, but in areas where mental health care is provided, officers on patrol should be particularly alert to persons who appear confused.

Officers who respond to such a patient-assistance call are considered support personnel and should always act under the direction of the caregiver. Security should not be expected to take over when a patient is out of control, a situation that calls for a team effort. It is very important that a caregiver and a security officer have a clear understanding of their respective roles, which should be formalized and practiced by both in training exercises. At the conclusion of an episode, the involved parties should jointly review all actions and reactions, either confirming or suggesting modification of the relevant security policies.

A patient being treated for a psychiatric problem who is leaving the facility against medical advice but in accordance with his or her rights may be rational but still in some danger. A psychiatric patient who turns up missing is something else entirely. The missing person may be a kidnap victim, someone who has feigned illness or injury to receive certain treatment, someone in an irrational state, or a patient who has simply decided to leave the hospital for whatever reason without telling anyone. This last situation is often referred to as a "patient elopement." (Note that in many emergency departments, patients fed up with long waits often leave without ever being seen by a caregiver; unless they are clearly incompetent, dangerous, or under forensic restrictions, a security alert may not be necessary in these situations.)

In any case, the missing patient must be immediately and thoroughly investigated, a joint responsibility of security and the staff of the unit. The first step is an exhaustive search, which may go beyond the property lines of the facility. Security personnel should be deployed as rapidly as possible to external points of the facility grounds; it is extremely important for security to search from the external points inward, while caregivers begin searching from the most internal point outward.

The need for a thorough search is illustrated by an incident that occurred in a Tennessee hospital. Four days after being admitted to the hospital's seventh floor for a stomach ailment, a 70-year-old woman was discovered missing. Only after an employee reported a foul odor two weeks later was her body discovered on the unfinished tenth floor, which was used for old furniture and medical records storage; the woman had apparently become confused and wandered off the unit on her own.

If there is any reason to believe that the patient has already left the premises and may be in danger due to his or her medical condition, the search by security should immediately be extended beyond the facility property as far as seems reasonable. At this point, too, the police should be notified.

The proper role of security is to locate the patient and coordinate his or her return to the treatment unit, by ambulance and after summoning assistance if the person is uncooperative. If the person refuses to wait and is either irrational or in immediate medical danger, the security officer must make a quick assessment of the need for physical restraint until help arrives, either holding or handcuffing the person as seems justified. There are obvious public relations, patient rights, and even legal ramifications to restraint procedures, thus as little force as possible should be used; but patients who are behaving in a way that presents a danger to self or others must be controlled.

■ *Patients Who Are Prisoners*

The patient who is also a prisoner and the patient who is brought to the hospital by police but has not yet been arrested both pose distinct threats. Such patients cause injuries, deaths, and destruction daily in the nation's health care treatment facilities.

Prisoner patients can be divided into two distinct categories: those being transported from a prison facility to the hospital for either outpatient or inpatient treatment, whose medical condition and propensity for violence or escape are already known; and those who have just been arrested and are in need of emergency medical care, who are more of a question mark. Prisoners in the second category may have been injured during arrest; may manifest signs of extreme stress, such as hypertension or heart attack; or may have swallowed a toxic or illegal substance inadvertently or deliberately. Although these prisoners may appear to present the greatest potential for danger, both types should be treated with equal caution. The patient who is coming directly from prison has had time to plan his or her actions; in fact, the medical need may itself be a ruse. An escape or attempted escape is not the direct responsibility of the hospital; it is the events that take place during the escape that can affect the facility, placing not only staff but other patients and visitors in jeopardy.

Patients who come in under police auspices but have had no charges filed against them, whether they appear to be suspects or victims of a crime, are an unknown quantity and should be considered as potentially very dangerous.

A major contributor to violence involving prisoner patients is the dichotomy such people present to law enforcement and medical personnel, who may have very different objectives and views of the situation. Intent on rendering confidential care that respects the patient's rights, the caregiver often assumes a superior role, demanding that certain custody and control measures be abandoned—that, for example, physical restraints be removed, and that police be excluded from treatment rooms. These demands may or may not be necessary or prudent. The custody and control procedures may or may not be unduly interfering with medical treatment. Clearly, protocols and expectations on all sides should be worked out in advance and not debated in the heat of the moment.

In one case, a prisoner patient removed the weapon from a police officer's holster. A nurse was able to gain control of the weapon before any harm was done, but the hospital later determined not to allow officers into the emergency department with their weapons. The reaction by the police was to take patients elsewhere for treatment and request that the hospital "please not call us to respond to situations in the emergency department." Eventually, a compromise was worked out: The police agreed to reassess their training, equipment, and procedures, and the hospital installed gun lockers for the temporary storage of officers' weapons in situations where they feel having a gun accessible is necessary.

◼ *Outpatient Clinics and Satellite Facilities*

The increased volume of outpatient treatment, especially in the clinic setting, has resulted in an increase in clinic-related security incidents. It is not hard to understand why. Clinic patients are often forced to wait for long periods to receive treatment, especially at peak demand times. They are often accompanied by family members and friends, including children needing special attention. There may be disappointments and disagreements over workers' compensation disability claims and fitness-for-duty evaluations. Waiting areas can become crowded and hectic, even loud and boisterous, creating an environment ripe for acting out.

The same security precautions, procedures, and controls used in the emergency department are basically applicable to the clinic environment. These include controlling access to treatment areas, maintaining good communications with the patient and persons accompanying the patient, and being alert for behaviors likely to escalate.

Where industry trends toward consolidation and decentralization converge, new demands are being placed on hospital security by the proliferation of treatment and support centers, which in the case of some health care systems today may be spread over an entire city. The result is a growing use in decentralized facilities of mobile security patrol checks, staff education in security principles and precautions, intrusion and panic alarms, and, when necessary, on-site security coverage. The explosion in home health care presents other new challenges, including the need for caregiver escorts in high crime areas and at night, advanced security awareness training for medical and support staff, and even self-defense training.

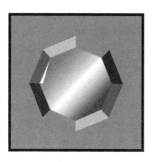

Conclusion

The approach of the millenium finds health care security in the midst of a paradigm shift, most notably toward decentralization and greater responsibility for security functions at the grass roots level.

In this new paradigm, the security department will become a resource to guide, direct, and support the individual operating units as they carry out their security responsibilities, while continuing to function as first responder to security incidents and coordinator of overall security systems. The security department also will provide security education and training throughout the organization.

Inevitably, this will mean a downsizing of security staffs and budgets and, as a consequence, greater reliance on electronic security equipment in the strategic security plan. What it must not mean is a loosening of standards and practices associated with a safe and secure health care environment.

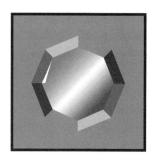

References

1. Trombly, T. 1995. Commentary: An epidemic of workplace violence. *Forum* 15:2, Winter.

2. Poster, E, Ryan, C. 1994. A multiregional study of nurses' beliefs and attitudes about work safety and patient assault. *Hospital Community Psychiatry* 45:1104–8.

3. Pane, G., Salness, K., and Winiarski, A. 1991. Aggression directed toward emergency department staff at a university teaching hospital. *Ann Emerg Med* 20(3):283–86, Mar.

4. Pesquera, A. 1994. Violence bursts into the nation's emergency rooms. *Denver Post* p 25A, Oct. 7.

5. Lehrman, S. 1994. Gunshot victims keep coming back. *Rocky Mountain News* p 58A, Dec. 1.

6. Calfee, B. 1989. Confidentiality and disclosure of medical information. *Nurs Management* 29:20, Dec. 29.

7. *The Security Advisor.* 1994. Annual report on animal rights incidents reveal increasing law-breaking violence. Aug. 17.

Index

Note: Page numbers followed by *f* indicate figures.